Coping with
PERIODS

Dr Judy Bury, the General Editor of this series, has worked in general practice and family planning for many years. She writes regularly on medical topics, and has a particular interest in self-help approaches to health care.

Other titles in the series include:
Coping with Caesarean and Other Difficult Births
Coping with Aging Parents
Coping with a Dying Relative
Coping with Sexual Relationships
Coping with Skin and Hair Problems
Coping with Your Handicapped Child

Coping with PERIODS

DIANA SANDERS

With a Foreword by
JILL RAKUSEN

Chambers

© Diana Sanders, 1985

Published by W & R Chambers Ltd Edinburgh

All rights reserved. No part of this publication may be reproduced, stored in a retrieval system, or transmitted, in any form or by any means, electronic, mechanical, photocopying, recording or otherwise, without the prior permission of W & R Chambers Ltd.

Illustrations by Sara Hills and Alison Johnston

ISBN 0 550 20503 9

British Library Cataloguing in Publication Data

Sanders, Diana
    Coping with periods.
    1. Menstruation
    I. Title
    612'.662   QP263
    ISBN 0-550-20503-9

Printed by Clark Constable, Edinburgh, London, Melbourne

Contents

INTRODUCTION	1
1. THE BIOLOGY OF PERIODS	3
2. YOUR OWN MENSTRUAL CYCLE	13
3. MANAGING PERIODS	19
4. PROBLEMS WITH PERIODS	28
5. PERIOD PAINS	36
6. PREMENSTRUAL TENSION	48
7. HELP FOR PERIOD PROBLEMS	67
8. HELPING YOURSELF WITH PERIOD PROBLEMS	72
APPENDIX	78

Dr Diana Sanders became interested while studying psychology, in the effects of hormones on women's moods. This led to a study of periods and premenstrual tension, and she spent a year in New Zealand, working on medical and self-help approaches to premenstrual tension. She now works as Research Officer in the Department of Community Medicine and General Practice in Oxford, but maintains her commitment to women's health issues. She also practises and teaches yoga.

Foreword

You may be wondering why another book about periods. There are quite a few already, and women nowadays know all about it—or all they wish to know. Well, maybe some women do know all they need, though fewer, I suspect, are completely happy about the state of their knowledge (or ignorance). And of those who have 'period problems', even fewer, I submit, feel completely happy with what they, or their doctors, do about these problems.

This book is one of the most helpful books I've read on the subject—and I've read quite a lot! It's also written by someone who herself acknowledges her own period problems and this contributes to the book's greatest strength: its respect for you, the reader. The book has many other strengths too. In the best feminist tradition, Diana Sanders combines sharing her experiences—and that of other women—with research and expertise developed over many years. She has produced a carefully researched, thoughtful, readable, and above all, practical book.

It examines a wide variety of approaches to period problems—not just the usual medical ones—and other issues as well. It recognises that we're all unique, that we're not all 'able-bodied', that we can learn a lot from ourselves and other women, and that how we experience menstruation is not only affected by what happens inside our bodies and minds, but also what's happening outside them too. In other words, the book takes a holistic approach.

For me, it's particularly gratifying to read a book by someone who is prepared to say that not even the experts fully understand menstruation—though you can be forgiven for thinking they'd got it all sewn up long ago—and also to see the care with which the author discusses the facts: when it comes to health and medicine, as with many aspects of life in general, there is rarely a simple answer to the questions we have. We at the Women's Health Information Centre believe in encouraging the production of health information for women that is responsible, helpful, respectful and honest. I think this book fits the bill.

Jill Rakusen
Women's Health Information Centre
1985

Preface

This book has arisen from several years of thought and research on an important area of women's health: Periods. When I started working on the menstrual cycle and premenstrual tension, in 1977, I was struck by the lack of information available about the basic biology of periods, the causes of common problems, and, most importantly, what women could do about difficulties with periods. Coping with periods was a subject only scantily covered in medical textbooks, not generally accessible to most women. Most treatments involved hormones and drugs, which are not always appropriate or effective. I started to ask questions: What can we do to help ourselves with problems and to help ourselves be healthy? The search for the answers led me through conventional science and medicine to alternative healers, folklore and herbalism, yoga, relaxation, massage, meditation, and a common-sense approach to nutrition and exercise. All these have something to offer towards solving problems and promoting health. As the information accumulated, I compiled it first as leaflets and pamphlets and finally as this book. My wish is for a variety of approaches to health to be accessible to all women, not just to those with access to specialist information or medical libraries. During my search for remedies for period problems, I personally have benefited from many of the approaches to health, and I appreciate the efforts and rewards of helping oneself to become healthy.

This book on 'self-help' could not have been written without the help of many people, whom I would like to thank warmly. Many women, in Britain and New Zealand, have shared their problems and remedies with me; I am especially grateful to those who have willingly taken part in my research in Edinburgh and Christchurch. For advice and information, I would like to thank Edinburgh Women's Advisory Group;

The Health Alternatives for Women (Christchurch, New Zealand); Hecate (Wellington, New Zealand); New Zealand Women's Health Network; The Women's Health Information Centre (London); Johanna O'Connor for her excellent advice on yoga; M. Brush for advice on premenstrual tension; and Anne McIntyre for her herbal knowledge.

Thanks to Elizabeth Gutteridge, the Berries at Holly Road, and the women at Karuna Falls for their contributions; and to my parents, Barbara Sanders and John Sanders, for endless support during the months of writing. Special thanks to Mary Houston, my friend, for discussion and comments on numerous drafts and for support in the processes of 'self-help'. I am grateful to the Psychology Department, University of Christchurch, New Zealand, where I was able to continue my research and compile this book. My helpers are but sources of inspiration and knowledge; I, as the writer, hold full responsibility for the contents of *Coping with Periods*.

Diana J. Sanders
Oxford, September 1985

Introduction

Coping with Periods is a guide to normal healthy periods and possible problems. It provides information to enable you to understand your periods. It will help you to deal with absent or irregular periods, heavy periods, painful periods and premenstrual tension.

Information about the basic biology of periods is not easily available and many of us are not really sure how our body works. So the first two chapters cover some simple biology and explain how to observe your own menstrual cycle and periods. Much of the information about common problems with periods is in medical textbooks and is not accessible to us. We may not recognise that we have a problem which could improve with help. Alternatively, we may leave it up to the doctor to recognise and treat problems such as painful periods or premenstrual tension. Doctors often recommend drugs to deal with our symptoms. We may leave the surgery not feeling quite sure about what is causing the problem or why we are given a certain treatment. Many women do not really like taking drugs or find that they are not always helpful. The chapters on period problems emphasise what you can do to help yourself: 'self-help'. For each problem there is a range of remedies you can try out so you can make an informed choice about helping yourself. You may need to experiment to find out what helps you, as we are all unique.

Obviously, not all problems are best dealt with by yourself. In some cases self-help is not advisable and you need expert advice, diagnosis and treatment. I have stressed when you *should* see your doctor. Some women prefer to try medical treatments, perhaps finding their problems too difficult to deal with by themselves. For each problem, there is a section on treatments available from the doctor. Chapter Seven is a guide to seeking expert help: how to talk to your doctor or see another doctor, and what alternatives there are to conventional medicine, if you would like to try another approach. Period problems might be an indication that your general health is not as good as it might be. Chapter Eight gives some hints on how to improve your health. Some women find that making sure that they are as healthy as they can be also solves period problems. Looking after yourself is a good starting place to coping with periods.

1. The Biology Of Periods

Every woman is aware of one obvious part of her menstrual cycle: periods or monthly bleeding, technically known as *menstruation*. Periods have many other names, too:

Common names for periods

The Curse	Travelling the Red Road
The Time of the Month	The Time of Flower
The Monthlies	My Red Aunt is Visiting
Having a Red Letter Day	The Magnificent Marquis
Taking my Period	is Visiting

Periods are only one part of a complex series of changes in our bodies during the menstrual cycle. The menstrual cycle is quite complicated and not properly understood, even by 'experts'. It is not surprising, then, that many women do not know much about how their bodies work and are mystified by the technical terms to do with the menstrual cycle.

But in fact the basic biology is really quite simple. It is important to understand the facts about our periods so we are in a better position to understand what goes wrong if problems do occur.

The Menstrual Cycle

The menstrual cycle is the name given to all the changes occurring in a woman's body each month in order to produce eggs and support a pregnancy if one should occur. The cycle involves processes to (a) release a ripe egg or *ovum* from one of the two *ovaries* and (b) prepare the body for an egg which has been fertilised by a sperm to grow into a *fetus*—the name given to a baby before it is born. The fertilised egg implants into the lining of the womb, the *endometrium*, where it grows for nine months. But if the egg is not fertilised and a pregnancy is not

Periods

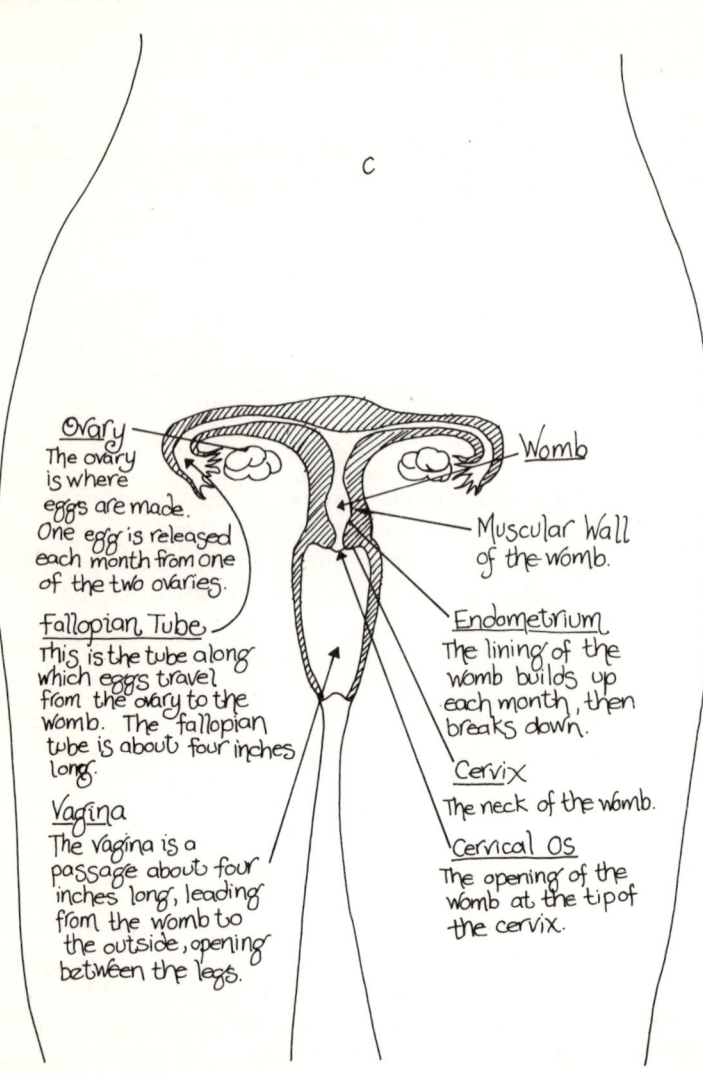

started during the menstrual cycle, the lining of the womb is shed. This is the period or *menstruation* and is usually the most obvious sign that the processes involved in the menstrual cycle are happening inside our bodies.

Hormones

The menstrual cycle is controlled by *hormones*. Hormones can be thought of as 'chemical messengers'. Along with nerves, they form part of our internal communication system, whereby different parts of the body signal messages to each other. There are two main types of hormones involved in the menstrual cycle: *Oestrogens* and *Progesterone*. These are made in the ovaries, and are controlled by hormones made in two glands in the brain: the *Hypothalamus* and the *Pituitary gland*.

Oestrogens are very important hormones for women because they make us female physically. They are responsible for the rounded contours of women's bodies and for hair in the pubic area and armpits. These hormones cause the development, growth and general 'upkeep' of the *reproductive system*: the womb, vagina, genitals and breasts. Oestrogens cause the lining of the womb to grow and develop ready for a fertilised egg to grow there. Progesterone also causes the womb lining to develop and it affects other parts of the body. For example, progesterone prepares the breasts to produce milk if a pregnancy starts. It causes the body temperature to rise slightly in the second part of the cycle.

Ovaries, Hormones and Wombs

The menstrual cycle can be thought of as three cycles, all happening at the same time. Firstly, the *cycle of the ovary*, where an egg develops and is released each month. Secondly, the *changing levels of hormones* which control the cycle. Thirdly, the *changes in the womb*, when the lining builds up and breaks down. These three cycles all take about one month, the time from one period to the next. They are shown in the next illustration.

First, the cycle of events in the ovary. In the first part of the

Periods

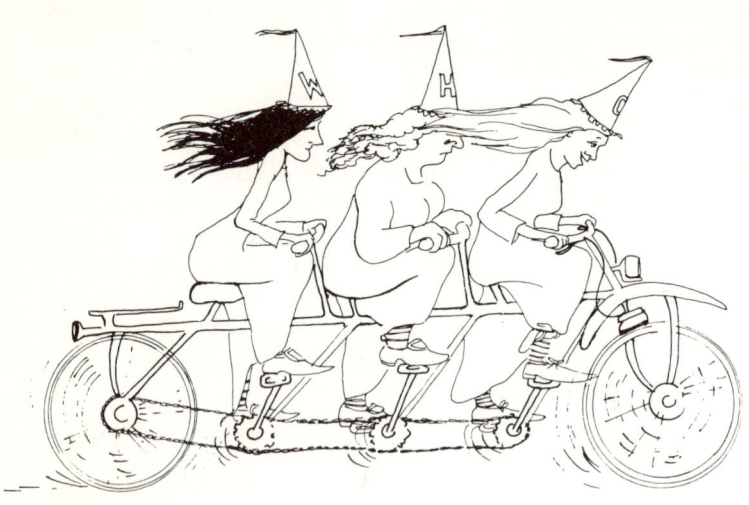

cycle, from the start of one period to ovulation (Day 1 to Day 14 in the illustration, p.7) egg-producing *follicles* develop in one of the two ovaries. The growing follicles produce oestrogens. During the later days of the first part of the cycle, one follicle develops more than the rest. No-one is quite sure how this one follicle is singled out as the one destined to ovulate. About the middle of the cycle (Day 14 in the illustration), when the developed follicle is ripe, it bursts and releases its egg. This is called *ovulation*. The released egg then starts its journey down the fallopian tube. If you have had intercourse and there are sperm in the fallopian tubes, a sperm might fertilise the egg. After ovulation, the empty follicle turns into a *corpus luteum* or yellow body, so called because it looks like a small yellow mass on the ovary. The corpus luteum produces oestrogens and progesterone. About one week after ovulation, if the egg has not been fertilised, the corpus luteum stops producing its hormones and it shrinks in size.

The Biology of Periods

These changes in the ovary cause the cycle of hormones shown in the illustration. Before ovulation, only oestrogens are produced by the follicles in the ovary. The amount of oestrogens increases, reaching a peak just before ovulation. After ovulation, both oestrogens and progesterone are made in the ovary so the amount of these hormones increases, reaching a high point about one week after ovulation. If the egg was not fertilised by a sperm and the corpus luteum begins to shrink, so the amount of oestrogens and progesterone starts to drop gradually in the week before the period.

This cycle of hormones affects the cycle of the womb. During the menstrual cycle the lining of the womb changes so that, if necessary, it can provide a place for a fertilised egg to grow and develop into a fetus. In the very early days of a pregnancy, the womb lining is the principal caretaker and provides all the blood and food supply for the growing baby. Later, the placenta develops to nourish the fetus. Before ovulation, oestrogens cause the womb lining to develop and grow. Tiny blood vessels and glands develop and the lining thickens. After ovulation both progesterone and oestrogens cause the lining to grow and thicken even more. In a

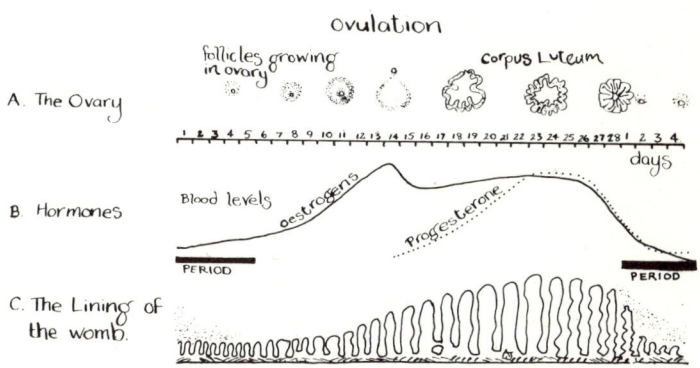

menstrual cycle in which the egg is not fertilised and you do not become pregnant, the fall in hormones in the last week or so of the cycle means that the thickened lining is not getting enough support from hormones and it can no longer survive. The lining begins to break down and is sloughed off. This is the period. The period signals both the end of one menstrual cycle and the beginning of the next.

Facts about the Normal Menstrual Cycle

How long is the menstrual cycle?

It is often believed that the time from one period to the next is a fixed twenty-eight days. In fact, periods are usually less predictable: most women have their periods at intervals of twenty-one to forty days. It is thought that the time from ovulation to the start of the period is fairly constant, about fourteen days. The first part of the cycle, from the beginning of a period until ovulation, is more variable.

Do we ovulate every month?

No: women may not produce eggs in up to 10 per cent of their menstrual cycles. Cycles without ovulation—technically called *anovulatory cycles*—are most frequent just after menarche (when periods start during puberty) and near the time when periods stop at the menopause. Cycles without ovulation may appear to be very similar to cycles in which an egg is produced, although they may be longer. If you do not ovulate, no progesterone is made in the second part of the cycle. This means that the effects of progesterone described above, such as breast tenderness and the rise in temperature, do not occur. Also, periods are usually painless if you do not ovulate.

Menarche and menstrual cycles in younger women

The start of periods is called the *menarche*. Before the first period, breasts develop, hair grows in the pubic area and armpits, and the body begins to change shape as fat is laid

The Biology of Periods

down in the hips, thighs and breasts. Menarche generally happens around 11-14 years, although any time from 9-16 years is quite normal. Girls are having their first periods at a younger age nowadays, compared to fifty years ago. This is probably due to better nutrition. The first few cycles tend to be long with unpredictable gaps between periods. Periods tend to stabilise and become more regular after the first few months or so.

The menopause

The end of a woman's periods is called the *menopause*. We reach the menopause around 46-52 years although any time between 40 and 60 is normal. The average age of the menopause has increased in the last fifty years, again probably due to improved nutrition. In the four years or so before the menopause, women often have irregular or erratic periods, with changes in the usual time between periods.

The pill and injectable contraceptive

The hormones in the *Combined Oral Contraceptive Pill*, oestrogen and progestogen, change the delicate hormone balance of the normal menstrual cycle so that no egg is released from the ovaries. The *Triphasic Combined Oral Contraceptive Pill* also contains oestrogen and progestogen, but the hormone content of the pills varies throughout the pill cycle, to mimic the normal menstrual cycle. Women on a combined pill should have some bleeding during the six or seven pill-free days: the pills' hormones cause the womb lining to build up slightly, and stopping the pill means that the lining is shed. But, strictly speaking, this is not a period in the usual way, but is called a pill withdrawal bleed. The blood loss may be lighter than usual, and period pains may be reduced. You may have some spotting or bleeding on days when you take the pill during the first two pill months, especially on low-dose pills: this 'breakthrough bleeding' seems to be less common on triphasic pills.

The *Progestogen-Only, or 'Mini', Pill* does not always prevent ovulation, but causes changes that make it difficult for sperm

Periods

to enter the womb, or for a fertilised egg to implant in the womb. It is fairly common for women taking the progestogen-only pill to have irregular periods which are sometimes more frequent than usual—perhaps two or three days bleeding twice a month—or sometimes later than usual. Occasionally, you may miss a period.

The *Injectable Contraceptive, Depo Provera*, involves injection of the hormone progestogen into a muscle where it is gradually absorbed into the body over two or three months. It acts in a similar way to the progestogen-only pill, and also stops ovulation. Generally, periods become irregular, or may disappear for a while. Periods may be disturbed for about six months after an injection, or longer for some women. Fertility may not return for eight to ten months, sometimes much longer.

How Bodies Change during the Menstrual Cycle

Our bodies are affected by the hormones involved in the menstrual cycle. This means that many parts of the body change during the cycle, along with the changes in hormones. Some of these fluctuations are quite noticeable to us, whereas others go on without our being aware of them.

Breasts commonly change during the cycle. Some women notice that they become fuller, more tender and sensitive, perhaps feeling tingly, in the second part of the cycle after ovulation, and especially just before a period. The tiny veins on the surface of the breasts, usually hardly visible, may become more prominent. The area around the nipples may feel very sensitive. Progesterone causes the tiny milk-producing glands in the breasts to grow, giving a fibrous, lumpy feeling. This is why just before a period is a bad time to do your regular monthly breast examination to check for unusual lumps. After a period, the normal lumps disappear; so this is a good time to check for unusual lumps.

Body temperature fluctuates during the menstrual cycle. Just before ovulation, temperature falls slightly, then rises after ovulation, dropping again just before your period.

Changes in cervical mucus. The cervix, or neck of the womb, makes mucous secretions, fluids to keep the vagina and cervix healthy and moist and to protect against harmful bacteria and germs. If you have intercourse and sperm enters your vagina, the mucus allows the sperm to swim up inside the womb and so into the fallopian tubes, where one may meet and fertilise an egg. But the mucus only allows sperm through around ovulation, not at other times of the cycle. Around ovulation, mucus is clear and tacky and there is a lot of it. At other times it is thick and white, and its thickness makes it hard for sperm to swim through.

Pain at ovulation: Mittelschmerz. Very occasionally, women experience pain or discomfort low down in the abdomen around the time of ovulation. It is usually felt only on one side and lasts from a few hours to a day or two, and may be accompanied by bleeding or spotting, like a light period. No one really knows what causes pain at ovulation. It may be caused by spasms or contractions in the fallopian tubes or womb; or at ovulation, the broken follicle may bleed a little causing irritation and pain. The bleeding or spotting may be due to a slight drop in hormones around ovulation.

There are changes in the *balance of fluids and salt* in the body during the menstrual cycle. After ovulation fluid and salt tend to build up, causing a slightly puffy or bloated feeling, especially in the breasts, tummy, face, fingers and ankles. You may notice that you pass more water during periods and around ovulation, as you shed this extra fluid and salt.

The composition of the blood changes during the cycle. The quantity of platelets, parts of the blood responsible for clotting, drops before and during a period. This explains why some women bruise more easily at these times, especially on the forearms and thighs.

The pigmentation of the skin changes: before a period, freckles and other marks may suddenly appear around the eyes, mouth, forehead, nipples and tummy.

As well as all these physical changes, many women have a cyclical pattern to their *moods and emotions.* These mood

Periods

changes seem to be so common that they are probably a normal and healthy accompaniment to our biological menstrual cycles. Generally the time before a period is accompanied by more 'negative' moods, perhaps sadness, tiredness, anxiety and withdrawal, feeling less willing to deal with other people's demands; in contrast, at other times, you may feel lively and energetic, happy and creative.

Sexual feelings and sexual activities can go up and down with the cycle. Many women feel more sexual around their periods or around ovulation. At these times, sexual activities can be more enjoyable.

2. Your Own Menstrual Cycle

To begin the process of coping with periods, we need to know about and understand our own menstrual cycles. One way is to observe and study ourselves. If you have problems to cope with, self-observation will enable you to know how your body works in its unique ways, and to see if there are changes if you start some of the processes of 'coping' discussed in this book. If you are particularly interested in finding out more about your menstrual cycle, or if you have problems, then try out one or more of these methods of self-observation.

Menstrual Cycle Diary

A good start is to keep a diary, recording your periods, moods, physical health and sexual feelings, and events and activities in your life. An example of a diary is shown here. Record the dates of your periods, days of bleeding, and note any discomfort, cramps or backache. Note your moods, energy or feelings of tiredness, whether you feel sociable or withdrawn, whether you need a lot of sleep—in fact, anything that is important to you. Keep a record of how you are physically, noting any breast tenderness, headaches, feelings of swelling, rashes or skin disturbances, infections or illnesses.

Write down important events, what you are doing, and any special stresses or pressures. After a few months it is fascinating to look for any patterns. Can you see cycles in your physical and emotional feelings, related to the time of your period? Is that seemingly unpredictable day of sadness or energy actually occurring at the same time in relation to your periods? Or is it all governed by the day of the week, or by events at work or at home?

Periods

MENSTRUAL CYCLE DIARY
One month is filled in, as an example

Instructions   Use the code and add others of your own to indicate how you feel each day. Write down any extra comments about what you have been doing, events, activities etc.

Month	Day of Month
March 1986	6: Br, T; 7: Br, Sw, T; 8: Ap, Br, Sw, T; 9: He, PP; 10: He, PP; 11–14: Period; 16: H; 17: H; 18: H; 26: Sw, PP
Comments	26: Pains, sad, sick side
April 1986	1: D; 2: D, He, Br; 3: D, He, Br, Sw; 4: T, He, Br, Sw; 5: T, I; 6: PP; 7–10: Period; 12: H; 15: S; 16: S; 17: S
Comments	

Code (examples)

H	= Very Happy	I	= Irritable
E	= Energetic	Br	= Breast Tenderness
S	= Sexual	Sw	= Swelling, Bloating
Sl	= Change in Sleep	He	= Headache
Ap	= Change in Appetite	PP	= Period Pains
D	= Depression, Sadness	▨	= Period
T	= Tired, Lethargic		

Your Own Menstrual Cycle

MENSTRUAL CYCLE CHART
(Partly filled in as an example)

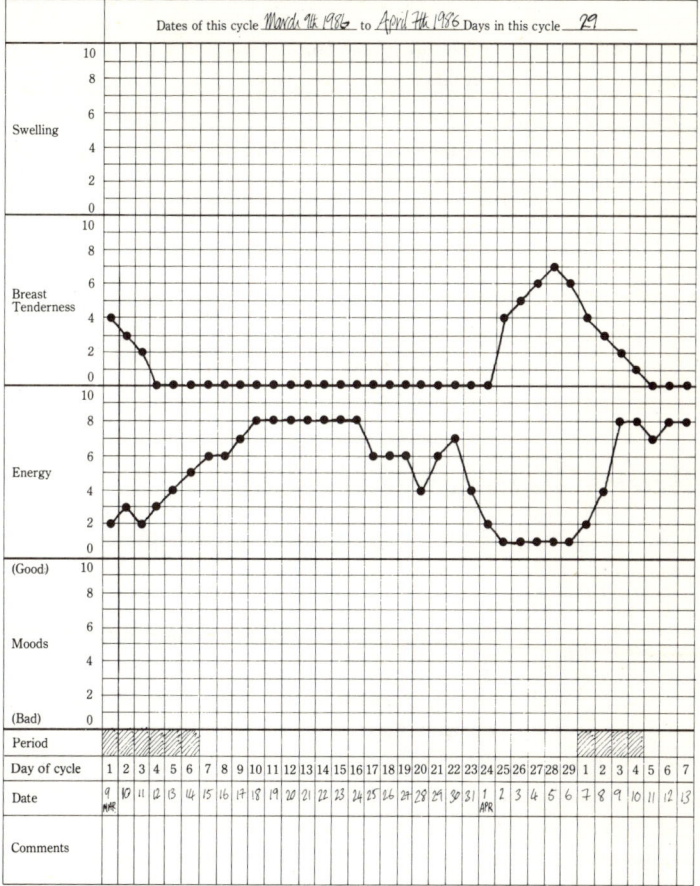

Periods

Chart of the Menstrual Cycle

Another way to record your moods and physical changes is to keep a chart, like the one on p.15. Write the date and day of your cycle along the bottom of the chart, with the first day of your period counting as day one. Up the side of the chart, various moods and physical feelings are represented as scales from 0 to 10, like the marks on a ruler. Each day, work out how much of each mood and physical feeling would best describe how you are that day. The amount will be between 0, which means none, and 10, which means a lot or severe. Then, put a mark on each scale. Leave a space for comments about events and activities.

Body Temperature Charts

Your temperature varies during the menstrual cycle. Try measuring your temperature each day for a few months to see if there is a pattern. Use an ordinary clinical thermometer, bought from a chemist, Family Planning Clinic or Well Woman Clinic. Take your temperature first thing in the morning, whilst still in bed and before going to the bathroom or drinking or eating anything or smoking. Leave the thermometer in place for at least two minutes. Record the temperature on a chart, like the one shown here.

Around the middle of the menstrual cycle, if your temperature drops slightly and then rises as in the completed chart, this probably indicates ovulation. If your temperature stays more or less constant and does not rise about two weeks before your period, this probably means that you did not ovulate in that cycle. But your temperature can be affected by many things, such as illness, tummy upsets, not sleeping properly, alcohol, taking various drugs and even sexual activity. So it is important to make a note of these in the space for 'comment' below the chart. Temperature charts are very useful for women who are trying to get pregnant to see whether and when they are ovulating.

Your Own Menstrual Cycle

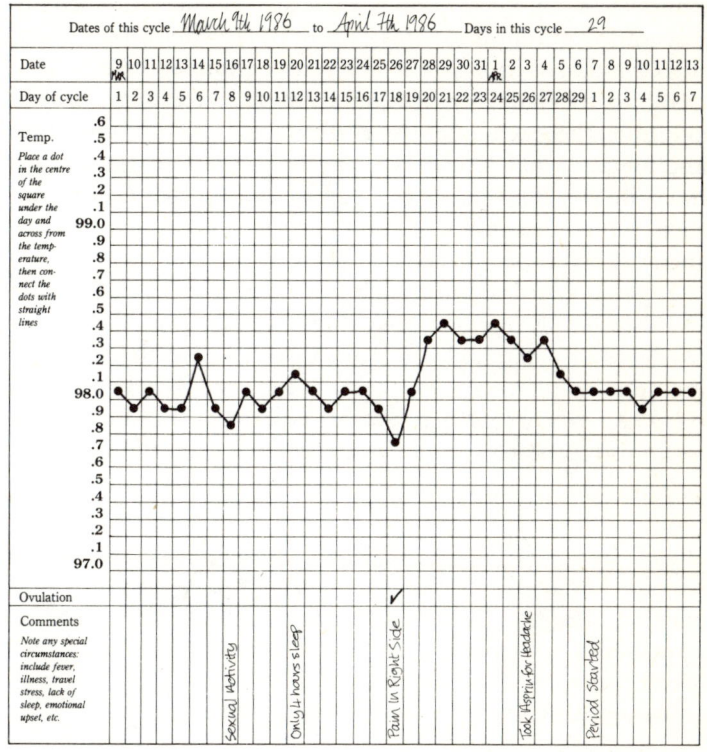

Changes in Cervical Mucus

Look for changes in the mucus from your cervix (neck of the womb) at different times of the cycle. Cervical mucus, combined with the secretions from the vagina, forms a moist discharge, present most of the time. Using your finger, scoop up some mucus from just inside your vagina, and examine it. Look at its quantity, composition and texture. Around ovulation there is a lot of cervical mucus. It is clear, glistening and slippery and stretches easily between your thumb and index finger. It looks like raw egg-white. At other times of the cycle, much less mucus is produced and it is thick, cloudy, sticky and will not stretch.

Keep a record of the changes in your mucus using a chart like this one. Keeping a note of changes in cervical mucus is the basis of a method of contraception called the 'Billings' method. Women with very regular menstrual cycles can find out when they are likely to ovulate and so know when either to avoid intercourse or to use contraceptive protection.

3. Managing Periods

Myths and Taboos about Periods

'Menstruating women should never salt pigs'

'Menstruating women must never enter a dairy or the butter will not churn, the cream will not rise, the cheese will not set'

'If you wash your hair while menstruating you will get brain fever'

'Menstruating women should not put their feet in cold water, or even their hands, in case it sends the blood to the head'

'Menstruating women should not go swimming'

A lot of myths and superstitions about periods arise from out-dated attitudes and beliefs based on ignorance. Previous generations thought that we shed 'bad blood' during our periods. But this is certainly not true. Our menstrual fluid is made of tissues and fluids that would have been used to nourish a new life if the egg had been fertilised. Your attitude to your body is important. You are more likely to feel tense and uncomfortable about your periods if you feel they are shameful or dirty. It is important to feel relaxed and good about periods so that everything can function in a healthy way. Periods can take up about one twelfth of your life, so it is a waste of valuable time to hide periods behind bathroom doors or limit yourself during periods. So don't listen to these myths about periods! Your own body is the best guide to what you can or cannot do. Some women like to withdraw during their periods and save strenuous activities for other times, whereas other women feel extra energetic. It is certainly not harmful to have baths or go swimming during periods. Hot baths may temporarily increase the menstrual flow and swimming in cold water may stop the flow for a while, but these are not harmful effects. Washing your hair will not affect your period. Exercise usually helps any discomfort during periods, so go for a run or play tennis if you feel like it.

A lot of taboos surround sexual activity during periods and some women feel uncomfortable about having intercourse whilst bleeding. But in fact, many women actually feel more sexually interested during a period. Despite this, they may feel uneasy about sexual activities with their partners. This may stem from fears that menstrual fluid is dirty, messy, smelly or even harmful. You may fear that your partner does not like the idea of sexual activity during your period. It helps to reassure yourself that periods are a natural, healthy part of being a woman. Talk it over with your partner, too, who may not be as worried by your periods as you fear.

Facts about Periods

Periods last, on average, between four and six days although they may be as short as two days or as long as eight.

Menstrual fluid is not pure blood, but contains mucus from the cervix and vagina and degenerated particles from the lining of the womb. The mixed content is not obvious because the blood stains the other parts.

During one period, women lose, on average, half a teacup of actual blood, although the other parts of the menstrual fluid make it seem like more.

Periods vary at different times. Close to menarche, in younger women, periods tend to be lighter, whereas older women approaching the menopause tend to have heavier periods. Periods can become heavier after childbirth or after coming off the oral contraceptive pill.

Emotional upsets, stress or changes in your life can lead to heavier or lighter periods, or episodes of heavy or prolonged bleeding.

The quantity of flow changes during the course of a period. 80 per cent of the total loss happens in the first two days.

Menstrual fluid itself does not smell. When it comes into contact with the air, it gets its characteristic smell.

What to do with the Menstrual Fluid

Fifty years ago women used pieces of cloth to catch their menstrual fluid. Today we have a variety of products to choose from, either sanitary pads or various forms of internal protection. When they first begin their periods, young women often prefer to use sanitary pads, trying internal protection later on. It is really up to the individual and there is no reason why you cannot use internal protection right from the first periods if you want to. The important thing is to find an appropriate, comfortable and convenient method of catching the menstrual fluid. You may have been using the same method of protection for years and feel quite satisfied with it. But you may like to try an alternative method of protection: there are several available.

Sanitary pads

There is a variety of pads to choose from. If you find the larger pads bulky and uncomfortable, try one of the brands of small but very absorbent pads. Pads can be used with a special belt, or are pinned to the underpants; or some have a sticky strip to fix to the underpants. Although there are deodorised pads available, the deodorant is unnecessary and could cause problems such as itchiness or a discharge.

Internal protection (Tampons)

Many women use tampons, but some have not been able to use them successfully. If you would like to try to use tampons, here are some guidelines:

A correctly-inserted tampon cannot fall out: it is held in place by the muscular vaginal walls. It cannot 'get lost', either, since the opening into the womb is far too small to allow a tampon through.

Some tampons come with an applicator. If you like to use applicators, it is best to use cardboard ones since there have been some worries about plastic applicators causing damage to the vagina.

It can help to use KY Jelly, a lubricant available from chemists, on the tampon or applicator, if your vagina is dry.

It can be a bit tricky to work out the best position for insertion: try squatting or raising one leg, and use a mirror to see what you are doing.

If in doubt, or having difficulty, seek 'expert' advice: mothers, sisters, friends, school teachers, school nurse, GP or nurse—in fact, most women— have been through the time of learning to use tampons.

Tampons and Toxic Shock Syndrome

Toxic Shock Syndrome (TSS) is an illness which occasionally affects women and which can be very serious. It may well be associated with the use of tampons. Although it quite a rare illness, many women use tampons, so it is useful to be aware of the symptoms and what precautions to take to avoid TSS. There are a variety of symptoms of TSS:

> A high fever which starts rapidly, with nausea and vomiting.
>
> Watery diarrhoea.
>
> Painful or tender muscles.
>
> Pain in the lower back or abdomen.
>
> Decrease in blood pressure, and sometimes shock.
>
> A rash, similar to sunburn, which may start 10 days or so after other symptoms start.
>
> Peeling skin, especially on the palms of the hands and soles of the feet.
>
> In its mild forms, TSS causes you to feel dizzy or off-colour.

The symptoms occur during or shortly after a period. Women with TSS have almost always been using tampons during the period, rather than other forms of protection. The symptoms of TSS seem to be caused by the poisons or toxins made by the bacterium *Staphylococcus aureus*, found in the vagina of women with TSS. *Staphylococcus aureus* is commonly carried on the skin and other parts of the body and is around all the time. Normally the bacteria do not get inside the vagina. We are usually resistant to any harmful effects. But some women using tampons are getting the bacteria into their vaginas. There, the bacteria multiply rapidly and make poisons which are quickly absorbed into the bloodstream, causing the symptoms of TSS.

No one is quite sure why this should happen to tampon users, although there are various theories. The bacteria may get into the vagina from the fingers whilst inserting a tampon. Normally the bacteria would not do any harm, but *Staphylococcus aureus* likes certain conditions in which to grow and make its toxins, especially dry places. It is possible that tampons dry the vagina too much so the bacteria can flourish there. Another theory is that tampons cause tiny scratches or ulcers in the vagina and bacteria get into the bloodstream through these. Plastic applicators, or possibly any kind of applicator, may slightly damage the vaginal walls.

Obviously, not all women who use tampons get symptoms of TSS. Many women have used tampons for years without any trouble at all. But it seems that new sorts of tampons are especially linked to TSS: tampons with plastic applicators and deodorised applicators; very absorbent tampons and the larger sizes; and the fact that manufacturers have changed the composition of tampons in the last few years, from all cotton to a blend of cotton and synthetic materials.

Here are suggested guidelines for tampon-users to minimise the risk of TSS:

Saturated tampons provide an excellent place for bacteria to grow. Change your tampon at least four times a day and, whenever possible, alternate their use with pads. This prevents the vagina becoming too dry.

Watch for vaginal dryness and irritation. If this happens, try using less absorbent tampons or, better, use other forms of protection for the rest of that period.

It is best not to use tampons if they cause you any pain or discomfort, especially when you are putting the tampon in or

Periods

pulling it out. Pain may indicate an abrasion or ulcer inside your vagina, caused by using tampons: the tampon may scratch the vaginal walls and this can lead to infection.

Be wary of tampons with applicators, especially the plastic applicators. Applicators may damage the vaginal walls.

Avoid deodorised tampons.

Whenever you can, avoid using tampons at night. Tampons can dry out the vagina if left in place for a long time.

Bacteria do not like cleanliness. Wash your hands before changing a tampon and bath or shower as often as you can during your period, ideally daily; if this is not possible, wash between your legs at least twice a day.

Avoid using tampons if you have any skin infections such as boils, abscesses, infected spots or impetigo, or infections around your nails. The bacteria causing these skin infections may also cause TSS. Wait until the skin infection clears up before using tampons.

If you feel ill or notice any unusual symptoms during your period, such as a fever, feeling dizzy or off colour, or feeling sick, it is important to get medical advice and treatment, since these may be early signs of TSS. Contact your doctor as soon as possible. Describe your symptoms and say whether you are having your period and using tampons. In its early stages TSS is treated with antibiotics. TSS can be very serious if not treated early on.

Diaphragms

A contraceptive diaphragm (or 'cap') can be used to collect the menstrual fluid. It holds more fluid than a pad or tampon and is also a cheap alternative to commercial pads and tampons. Remove the diaphragm when you think it is full; experiment to work out how often you need to empty it. Wash the diaphragm in water and reinsert it. Some women find diaphragms excellent although others find them a little messy, tending to leak if allowed to fill. They may be best for your lighter days, more absorbent protection being better for heavier days.

Natural sponges

Many women are using natural sponges as a means to soak up

Managing Periods

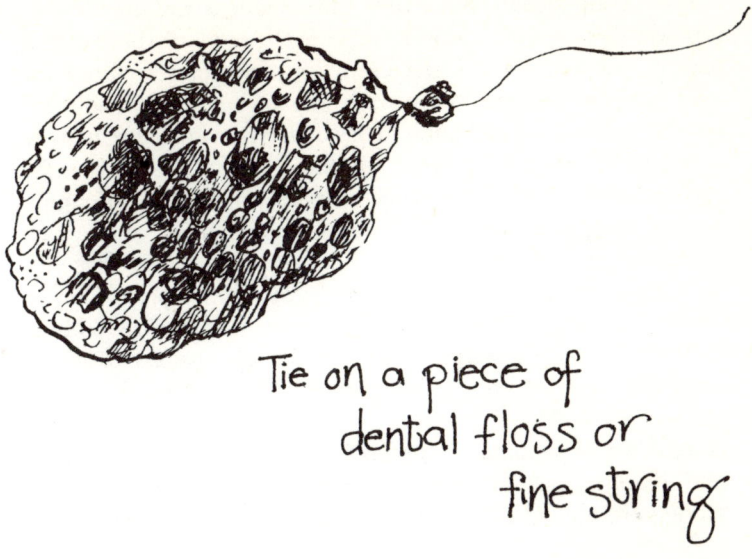

Tie on a piece of dental floss or fine string

the menstrual fluid. They are cheaper than tampons, more comfortable and are good for dry or sore vaginas. You can buy natural sponges at chemists and some health food shops. A piece of sponge, the size shown, absorbs as much as one regular size tampon or pad. Sponges with small holes absorb more than those with larger holes. Tie a piece of dental floss or fine string through one end of the sponge to help you to remove it (like a tampon), although you may prefer to remove the sponge using your fingers.

How to use a sponge: Dampen the sponge thoroughly, squeeze out the excess water and, using your fingers, push the sponge inside your vagina, leaving the string dangling out between your legs, like a tampon's string. To remove the sponge, either pull the string, as for removing a tampon, or insert two fingers into your vagina and pull the sponge out. Wash the sponge using warm water and pure, non-perfumed soap. Rinse and squeeze out the sponge and reinsert it. You may need to experiment to find out how often you need to wash your sponge: most women find they become saturated every three to five hours, varying according to how heavy the period is.

It is a good idea to have two or three sponges and use them in rotation during your period. Take a clean spare sponge in a plastic bag with you when there are not good facilities for washing your sponge. When you remove your sponge, squeeze out the excess fluid and pat it to dry on a tissue and store it away in the plastic bag until you can wash it out. Each sponge lasts for two or three periods. It is not necessary to sterilise it. Thoroughly reclean it by soaking for a few hours in a solution of one part white vinegar to three parts water; then let the sponge dry thoroughly in the air and store it ready for the next period. If you have a vaginal infection or sexually-transmitted disease (STD or VD) do not use the same sponge for the next period as it may carry the infection back to you the next time it is used.

Note: Very occasionally TSS has affected women using sponges and diaphragms. It may be best to follow the suggested guidelines (above) if you use any form of internal protection.

Periods and Disabled Women

If you are disabled you may have to cope with a number of special problems with managing periods. Some disabled women meet the following sorts of problems:

> Lack of suitable sanitary protection designed to meet the special needs of disabled women.
>
> Lack of suitable facilities for changing and disposing of sanitary protection and for washing during periods.
>
> Periods, especially heavy flow, can be a discomfort for women who spend much of the day sitting and who cannot use internal protection.
>
> Bulky pads can cause pressure sores and chafing, especially if not changed frequently.
>
> Women with impaired sensation around the vaginal area find it hard to recognise when pads and tampons are saturated and need changing.

Spills and leakages can not only be uncomfortable, but can increase the risk of vaginal infections, such as thrush.

There is a general lack of information about management of periods for disabled women and for those caring for them.

The Disabled Living Foundation has information about special aids and protective garments. Liberation Network is an organisation for disabled people. Their addresses are given at the end of this book.

4. Problems With Periods

Although most women have fairly normal, regular periods most of the time, certain situations arise that might interfere with your menstrual cycle or stop your periods for a while, or produce unusual patterns of bleeding. This chapter covers some of the common problems with the menstrual cycle and periods. The menstrual cycle is a delicately balanced system. Various things can easily throw the system out of balance for a while, leading to changes in your periods. What sort of factors influence the menstrual cycle?

Emotional upsets and stress

Emotional upsets and stress can produce at least a temporary change in your periods. A few cycles may become longer or shorter; your periods may become heavier or lighter, longer or shorter. You may miss a few periods or your periods may stop completely for a while. Stress need not necessarily be severe for your cycle to change or for your periods to stop. A change of occupation, moving house, going on holiday or family upsets can influence your periods. Some women are very sensitive to stress whereas others can weather the most devastating crises with no upsets to their systems.

Body weight and nutrition

Weight and eating habits play a part in the menstrual cycle and periods. In adolescence, we do not generally start having periods until reaching a certain body weight. Then, both losing and gaining weight can affect your cycle or periods. Women who lose a lot of weight through deliberate, severe dieting or vomiting almost always stop having periods. Women with erratic eating habits, sometimes eating a lot, sometimes hardly eating at all, often have erratic periods.

Problems with Periods

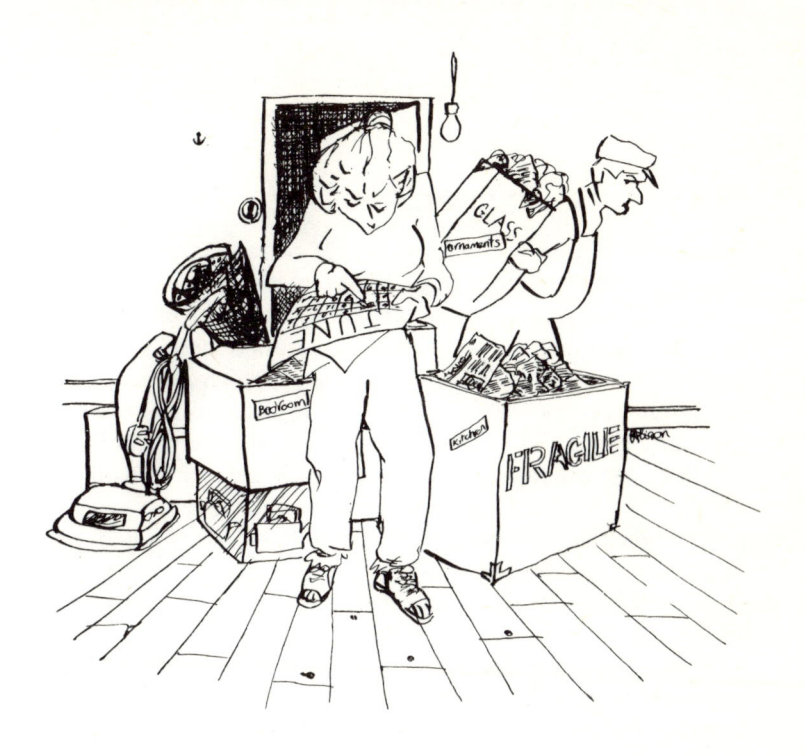

Exercise

Long-distance runners, athletes, gymnasts, dancers and swimmers undergoing rigorous and strenuous exercise programmes commonly have irregular periods; sometimes periods stop completely for a while. Milder exercise can also affect your menstrual cycle or periods, especially when you start to take more exercise than usual.

Other women

Women who live together or spend a lot of time together find that their cycles 'synchronise' so that they have their periods almost at the same time each month.

Common Problems with Periods and What to Do

No periods (Amenorrhoea)

Pregnancy and the menopause are the commonest reasons for women's periods to stop. But if your periods suddenly stop and you are definitely not pregnant or coming up to the menopause, there may be other causes. The most common reasons for your periods to stop are related to the things which influence the menstrual cycle described above. If you are under stresses or pressures, in the midst of emotional upsets, changing your life or routines, for example, your periods may stop for a while; a change of weight or starting a new or rigorous exercise programme may influence your periods. *Change* seems to be the key factor.

Apart from these common causes, a number of other things may stop your periods:

After a pregnancy, even if you are not breast-feeding, your periods may not return immediately. This can also happen after a miscarriage or termination of pregnancy (abortion).

Breast-feeding commonly and normally stops your periods. It may take a while for your periods to settle down again whilst weaning your baby off breast milk.

The combined and progesterone-only oral *contraceptive pill* and contraceptive injections (Depo Provera) may affect your bleeding, even after stopping the pill or injections.

Illnesses and drugs may stop your periods. If you are ill, or are recovering from an illness, or are taking drugs, and your periods stop, check with your doctor.

Accidents, injuries or operations, especially in the pelvic area—for example a contraceptive sterilisation—may stop your periods for a while.

Some *medical conditions* such as polycystic ovaries, can be the cause of persistent loss of periods. It is best to get advice and treatment for these.

What to do if your periods stop

Most of the time, it is usually fairly obvious why your periods have stopped. It may be because of changes in your life or routines; stress; emotional upsets; a recent change in weight; increased physical activity; illness. Usually when these factors are sorted out, or life becomes more settled, or you adjust to the changes in lifestyle, your periods return. Some women always lead fairly stressful and hectic lives, constantly changing their routines. No periods may, for some, be 'the norm' rather than a problem. In fact, during stress and change, it is good not to have periods: your body is directing energy into dealing with the stresses. In these cases, try not to be over-concerned or worried about not having periods. Try and sort out the stress or other causes rather than taking drugs to make your periods return. It may help to watch your general health and nutrition (see Chapter 7). If you are obviously over or under what is a good, healthy weight for you, it may help to change your weight through nutrition and exercise, especially if not having periods is worrying you.

Having no periods is more of a problem if you are trying to get pregnant, as it may indicate that you are not ovulating. In this case, if there is no obvious or easily-remedied cause for your lack of periods, it is a good idea to visit your doctor. You should have a full history taken and be given a physical examination including an internal examination. You can be referred to a specialist, usually a gynaecologist, to have your hormones and glands tested, by urine and blood tests and X-rays. You may be prescribed drugs to make you ovulate.

Irregular Periods

Some women's periods are always fairly unpredictable. This can be inconvenient, or a problem if you cannot tell quickly if you become pregnant. It can be a worry for women who are trying to get pregnant. Medically, periods which are irregular are not a cause for concern and are not treated unless you are seriously concerned about your fertility. However, if you normally have regular periods and you suddenly start to have periods at irregular times, especially if the length or heaviness of the period changes as well, this may suggest something is wrong. It is good to check this with your doctor. In the years just after the menarche and just before your periods stop at the menopause, irregular periods are fairly common; this may be because you do not ovulate during some of your menstrual cycles at these times. Stress and changes in life can make your periods temporarily less regular.

What to do to help regularise your periods

If your periods are irregular, try some of the suggestions for 'no periods' above: check to see whether any aspects of your lifestyle are influencing your periods. Think about stresses and changes, emotional upsets, exercise, weight and nutrition. Yoga might help (see Chapter 8): many women who take up yoga find that their periods settle down and become more regular.

Heavy Periods

Periods may be heavy in a number of ways. They may come regularly every month, but are either very heavy or very long, or perhaps both heavy and long. Or they may be heavy and irregular, coming perhaps after twenty-one days in one cycle and forty-eight days in the next. It is important to distinguish between regular and irregular heavy periods. If they are regular, this is generally due to an easily correctable cause, whereas if there is no pattern to the periods, it may be the first symptom of something wrong inside the womb. Bleeding patterns also vary a lot between women. Some women always have heavy periods, requiring frequent changes of pads or tampons, or perhaps lasting twelve days or so. The presence of large clots, which look like liver, in the menstrual fluid simply means that the bleeding is heavy; there is no other significance.

Heavy and/or long periods are more a cause for concern if they start suddenly and you previously had lighter and/or shorter periods—that is, if you notice a sudden *change*. What might cause your periods to change?

Problems with Periods

In the year or more leading up to the menopause, periods often change, becoming less regular, longer and heavier.

Emotional upsets and stress can cause heavy or long periods.

Coming off the pill may be followed by a few heavier periods.

The IUCD (coil or loop). This may make periods heavier and more painful, especially for the first few months after it is fitted and especially if you have never had a child. It is a fairly common side effect which usually settles down after a while. But check that the IUCD has not been dislodged. Feel for the string as instructed by the doctor or clinic who fitted the IUCD. If you cannot feel the string or if you can feel the plastic of the IUCD itself, go to your doctor. If your periods suddenly get much heavier or more painful, get the IUCD checked by the doctor. Very rarely, bleeding or pain may be due to the IUCD making its way through the wall of the womb.

There are various, more serious, reasons for your periods to change. These may cause pain with your periods as well as heavy bleeding. It is important to have these investigated by your doctor.

Fibroids. These are small, non-cancerous, tumours inside the womb, which can cause heavy periods which may be painful as well. They can be surgically removed. If they are causing very heavy periods (or severe pain), it is sometimes necessary to have a hysterectomy (surgical removal of the womb).

Endometriosis. This is an uncommon condition when small fragments of the lining of the womb start to grow outside the womb, such as on the ovaries, or inside the abdomen. When you have a

Periods

period, the fragments of womb lining also start to bleed, causing pain. Endometriosis is usually treated by taking hormones; sometimes the womb fragments can be removed by surgery.

Pelvic infection. This is sometimes called Pelvic Inflammatory Disease. It usually causes constant pain but can cause very painful periods and very heavy periods. Pelvic infection is more common if you have an IUCD in place, especially if you have never had children. Occasionally pelvic infection is due to VD, so it is important to go to a VD clinic if this may be the case. Pelvic infections are treated with antibiotics.

Early stages of womb or cervical cancers.

A hormone imbalance. If you are not making enough progesterone after ovulation, you may have heavy periods.

Sometimes doctors recommend an operation called a *Dilatation and Curettage*, or *'D & C'*. It is done in hospital under general anaesthetic. The cervix is gradually dilated (stretched) until a small spoon-shaped instrument, a curette, can be inserted. The inside of the womb is scraped and examined for possible causes of heavy bleeding. As well as being useful for diagnosing the cause of heavy periods, a D & C can occasionally cure heavy periods: after the operation, your periods may return to normal or become lighter.

For severe period problems, doctors sometimes advise a *hysterectomy*—surgical removal of the womb—especially if you are sure you do not want future pregnancies. Whilst a hysterectomy may be necessary for some severe conditions such as cancer, it is a major operation and there may be some alternative treatments that you can try first, such as hormones, prescribed by your doctor.

Self-help measures for heavy periods

So long as heavy periods are not caused by any of the more serious conditions described above, you can try some remedies yourself:

Iron deficiency can cause, as well as result from, heavy bleeding. Make sure your diet includes the iron-rich foods listed in Chapter 7. You may need additional iron supplements for a while if you are very run down or anaemic. These are available from chemists and health food shops, or on prescription from your GP. Vitamin C helps your body to absorb iron, so eat fresh fruit and vegetables, perhaps an orange every day, especially if you are taking iron supplements.

Calcium may help heavy periods. As for iron, check that your diet includes the good sources of calcium, listed in Chapter 7. You may need calcium supplements. It is best to take calcium with magnesium, as Dolomite, available from health food shops. Take it as directed on the packet.

Additional iodine may help: kelp, a seaweed, is a good source of iodine. You can buy kelp tablets from health food shops.

Recently, there have been some interesting links found between Vitamin A deficiency and heavy periods, especially with 'flooding'—sudden rapid gushes of menstrual fluid, containing clots. Make sure you include foods rich in Vitamin A (also listed in Chapter 7) in your daily diet.

Evening Primrose Oil, manufactured under the name 'Efamol', can help heavy and prolonged bleeding. You can buy Efamol from health food shops and chemists. The same regime taken for premenstrual tension (see Chapter 6) seems to help normalise heavy periods within two or three months.

5. Period Pains

Most women experience some discomfort with their periods at some time in their lives. Period pains or cramps are technically known as *dysmenorrhoea*. Period pains are usually felt in the lower abdomen and sometimes down the insides of the legs and in the lower back. The pain can be sharp and spasmodic, coming in waves, or it may be felt as a dull, continuous ache. It usually starts soon after the period starts, but sometimes the pain begins before the bleeding. A few women get period pains after the first day or two. Period pains last anything from a few hours to two to three days. Period pains may be accompanied by sickness or nausea, faintness, diarrhoea or constipation.

Period pains differ a lot between women. Some have no trouble at all and others have slight but manageable cramps. For some women period pains are severe and they feel so unwell and faint that they function below par, or occasionally need a day or two off work. Period pains also differ between periods. Most women say that some periods are better than others.

Who gets Period Pains and When?

Period pains are more common in younger women in their teens and early 20s than in the 30s upwards. They generally improve or disappear as you get older. There is a popularly held belief that the pains disappear after having a baby, but this is not always the case. Not all women do get relief after having children, and a few get worse pains. It is thought that period pains only occur if an egg is produced during the menstrual cycle. Women who do not ovulate, for example, shortly after the menarche, do not generally get period pains.

Sometimes cramps are worse when we are under stress or for a time after coming off the pill. Having an IUCD (loop or coil) fitted can make period pains worse for a while.

Causes of Period Pains

Period pains are usually caused by the normal biological processes involved in periods. During a period, to help the removal of its lining, the womb contracts slightly in a rhythmical way. Similar, but much stronger, contractions occur during labour. Period pains are caused by these contractions. Women with period pains seem to have particularly strong womb contractions at the start of their periods. The strong contractions cut off the supply of blood and oxygen to the muscles of the womb. As a result, the womb muscles cramp, just like cramps felt when any other muscles get tired. Hormones called *Prostaglandins* cause the womb to contract. Women who have painful periods have large amounts of prostaglandins in the womb. Prostaglandins may also cause the headaches, dizziness, sickness and diarrhoea which sometimes accompany period pains.

Other causes of period pains

Some medical problems can cause period pains. These include problems with an IUCD, fibroids, endometriosis and pelvic infection: see previous chapter. If you are in your 20s, 30s or 40s and your periods suddenly start to become painful for no apparent reason—you notice a change—*it is important to check with your doctor* for a medical cause.

Self-help for Period Pains

There are a number of different things that you can do to relieve period pains, listed below. Try one or a few to see what helps.

If you are trying to help yourself with period pains, it is good to *plan ahead*. Try and work out in advance when your period is due and how this might affect what you have to do. Before your period arrives, think about what you can do to help yourself, and perhaps practise some of the remedies or exercises. It would be good if women could plan schedules, meetings and important events so as not to have too much to do at the start of a period, but this is not always possible. Do what you can, though.

The remedies you can try include heat, hot drinks, herbs, relaxation, exercises, yoga, massage, orgasm, calcium, not smoking and painkillers.

Heat

Heat helps to relax your muscles and ease the pain. Try curling up with a hot-water-bottle, or have a warm bath. Put some aromatic bath oils or soothing herbs in the bath water: soak a handful of chamomile flowers or juniper needles in a pint of boiling water for twenty minutes and pour this into the bath water.

Hot Drinks and Herbs

Internal heat helps. Avoid tea and coffee if you can as the caffeine can irritate your stomach. Try a range of *herbal teas* instead. There are numerous herbs which women have traditionally used to relieve cramps (see Appendix), or herbal tablets are available from health food shops. A small amount of *alcohol* made into a hot drink with hot water, lemon and honey is a useful measure on occasions. Alcohol may improve the blood supply to the pelvis and increases your tolerance of pain. But too much alcohol can make you sick, dizzy or sleepy.

Relaxation

Since period pains are caused by muscles contracting, learning how to relax will help ease the pain. Also, relaxation helps make pain more tolerable, because you are not trying to resist or fight it. It is especially good to learn to relax if you tend to tense up during period pains, and want to curl up into a tight ball, clench your teeth and take short shallow breaths.

Here are three different relaxation exercises. Try them and find one that suits you. The first exercise is good to do when you have bad period pains, to help relieve the pain at the time. It helps you to relax your abdomen and pelvis and to breathe deeply so as to bring oxygen to your cramping muscles. The other two relaxation exercises can be done either during period pains or whenever you feel tense and in need of relaxation. Before relaxing take off your shoes and loosen tight clothes. When you finish a relaxation exercise, get up slowly and gently, keeping the feelings of relaxation even when you start doing other things.

1. Relaxation breathing

Lie down, on a bed or on the floor, with your head supported and a firm cushion under each knee, with your legs bent. Let go of tension in your body, especially concentrating on relaxing your pelvis and abdomen. As you count to five, breathe in deeply through your nose. Let your abdomen and chest expand as they slowly fill with air. Imagine the air filling your head, neck, arms, abdomen, pelvis and legs, replacing any tension. Then breathe out through your mouth, counting down from five to one. Try to push out all the air, keeping your body relaxed. Keep breathing regularly and repeat this ten times. When you are used to the exercise, count up to ten on each in breath and down from ten as you breathe out.

2. Tensing and relaxing

In this exercise you tense up and then relax different parts of your body until you feel completely relaxed. Sit in a comfortable armchair or an office chair with arms, so that your arms are supported and your head is resting either on the back of the chair or on a wall behind the chair. Have your feet resting comfortably on the floor. Breathe deeply and regularly whilst you do the exercise. When you are comfortable, start to tense and relax different parts. Start with your right hand. Tense up your hand into a tight fist, hold for five seconds, then let it go and allow your hand to relax for about ten seconds. Then, tense and relax your left hand in the same way.

You do this tension-relaxing sequence as follows:

1 Right hand
2 Left hand
3 Right arm
4 Left arm

5 Head, face, eyes, nose and mouth, especially your jaw
6 Shoulders and chest
7 Abdomen and pelvis
8 Right leg
9 Left leg
10 Right foot
11 Left foot

When you have tensed and relaxed each part of your body, sit for a few minutes feeling completely relaxed all over.

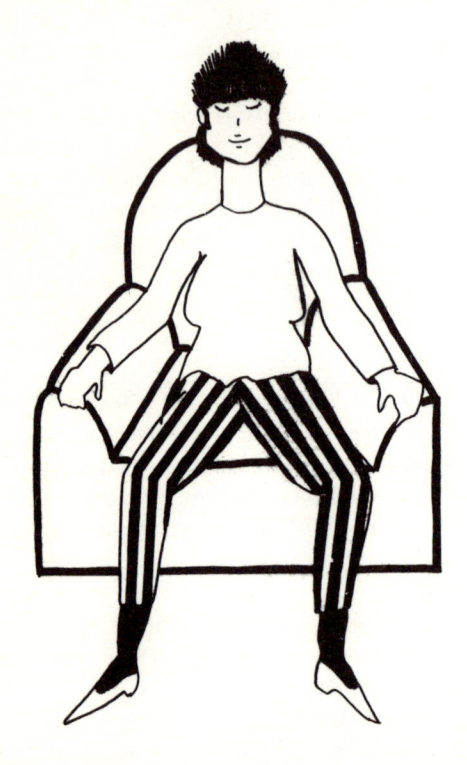

3. *Complete relaxation*

Lie down on your back on the floor or on a bed, making sure you are warm and comfortable. Rest your head on a cushion or put a pillow or folded blanket under your head and shoulders. When

Period Pains

you are comfortable, close your eyes and let all tension leave your body. Become aware of each part of you relaxing more and more each time you breathe out. Keep your mind on your body and try not to get distracted by other thoughts. Stay relaxing for ten minutes or so.

Exercises

Contrary to many myths and misconceptions, exercise during your period is not harmful. It helps to relax muscles, increasing the supply of blood and oxygen to your cramping womb, and so helps relieve pain.

Here are a few exercises which you can try. A short time spent doing exercises may relieve even severe cramps. Wear loose clothes when doing exercises. Undo any tight waistbands and remove your shoes.

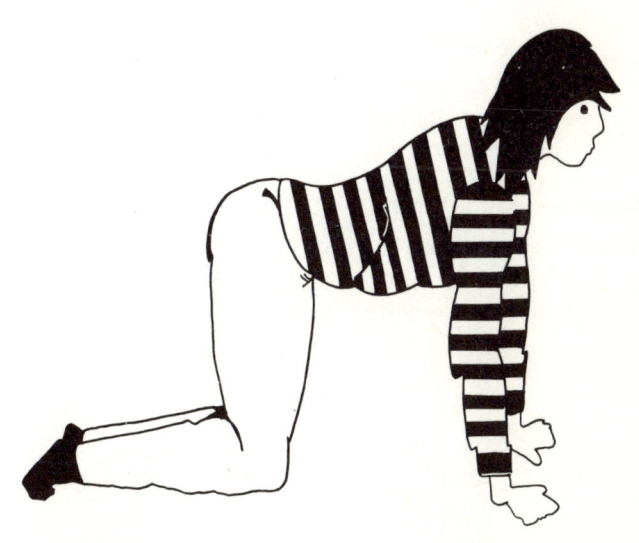

1. Cat stretch

Go down on all fours, placing your palms flat on the floor, keeping your shoulders down and make your back straight like a table (i). Breathe in slowly through your nose. Then, breathe out slowly and deeply, at the same time pulling in your abdominal muscles and humping your back up, looking

Periods

down towards your navel (ii). Hold this position for a count of five. Then let go and breathe in slowly through your nose, at the same time lifting your head to look upwards and arching your back so your abdomen moves downwards. Hold for a count of five. Repeat six times.

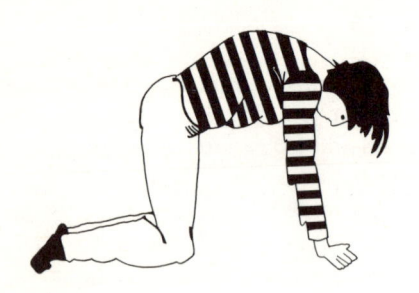

2. Dry land swimming

Put a pillow on a sturdy, strong coffee table or chair. Lie on your front on the pillow and put your hands on the floor in front of you to balance. Put your legs out straight behind you, horizontal to your body (Figure i). Now bend your knees so that your heels are pointing towards the ceiling. Next, spread your knees so that your thighs are apart (ii). Then, straighten your legs by first dropping your feet down so your legs are horizontal to your body then bringing your legs together until

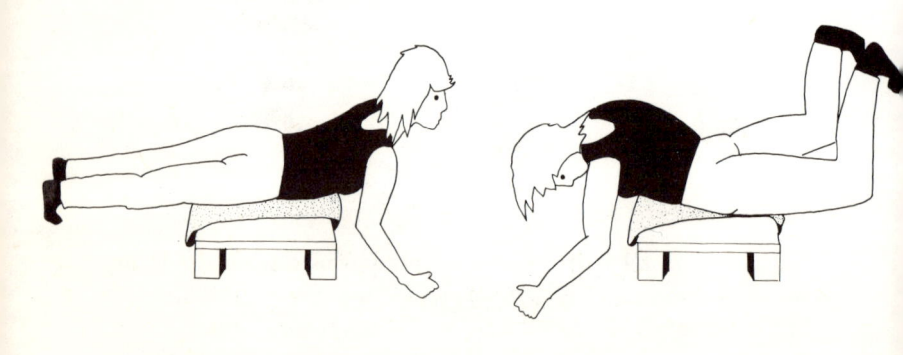

Period Pains

your knees touch. Start by doing this for two minutes; then gradually build up to six, resting every minute or so. It helps to do this exercise two or three days before your period as well as on the first day; the movements stimulate the blood supply to the pelvis.

3. The pelvic rock

Try a simple exercise of rocking your pelvis. It helps to stimulate the blood flow to your pelvis and womb. Standing up straight, put one hand on your lower tummy and the other hand on the small of your back. Push down with the hand on your back whilst you tighten your buttocks and lift up your abdomen with your pelvic muscles. Then, push down with the hand on your abdomen and lift your buttocks up so your pelvis tilts in the other direction. Gently rock your pelvis up and down for a minute or two, in a slow rhythm. After a while you will be able to do this without using your hands.

4. Child stretch

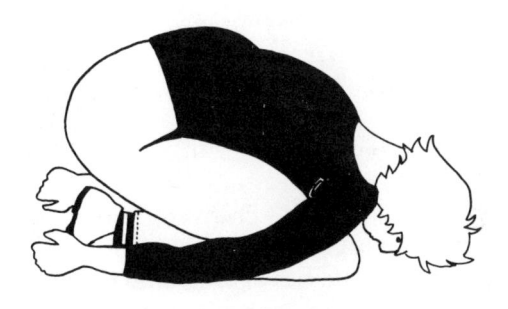

This exercise is also good for backache. Begin by sitting on your heels. Slowly stretch your body forward until your forehead touches the floor in front of you, stretching your tummy out over your bent legs. Either stretch your arms out in front of you or rest them alongside your body. Let your body relax down onto your legs and let your tummy go loose. Close your eyes and breathe slowly and deeply with a regular rhythm. Rest for a few minutes until you feel relaxed and the pain begins to ease.

More strenuous exercise can help period pains. If you have time and feel up to it, a brisk walk, a run, swimming or a game of tennis may help.

There may be times when period pains are very severe and you feel faint, weak and unwell. In this case, you may definitely feel that exercises are not appropriate. It may help to do some relaxation first (see above) and then do some gentle exercises after relaxing for a while. There are many other exercises which women have found useful for period pains. Some books are listed at the end of the book. Exercises for childbirth are also very effective for dealing with cramps. The National Childbirth Trust (their address is at the end) can provide further information.

Yoga

Many yoga poses or exercises are very good for relieving period pains. It is best to learn yoga in classes: it is more fun than learning on your own and you also learn the exercises correctly. If you would like to find out more about yoga, read the section on yoga in the Appendix, or have a look at the books listed at the end. If you cannot go to classes but would like to try some yoga on your own, a few exercises are described in the Appendix.

Orgasm

Having orgasms can very effectively relieve period pains. When you have an orgasm, lots of blood flows to your pelvic regions, helping the muscles of the womb to relax. It does not matter how you have an orgasm for it to work: either with your partner or on your own.

Period Pains

Calcium

Extra calcium might help your period pains. Try taking calcium in the week before your period and on the first day or two of bleeding. It is best to take calcium with magnesium, as Dolomite tablets, available from health food shops and chemists. Take it as directed on the packet.

Massage

Rubbing and massaging your pelvic area and lower back helps you to relax your pelvis. You can massage yourself or ask a friend or partner to lend a hand. Try using some

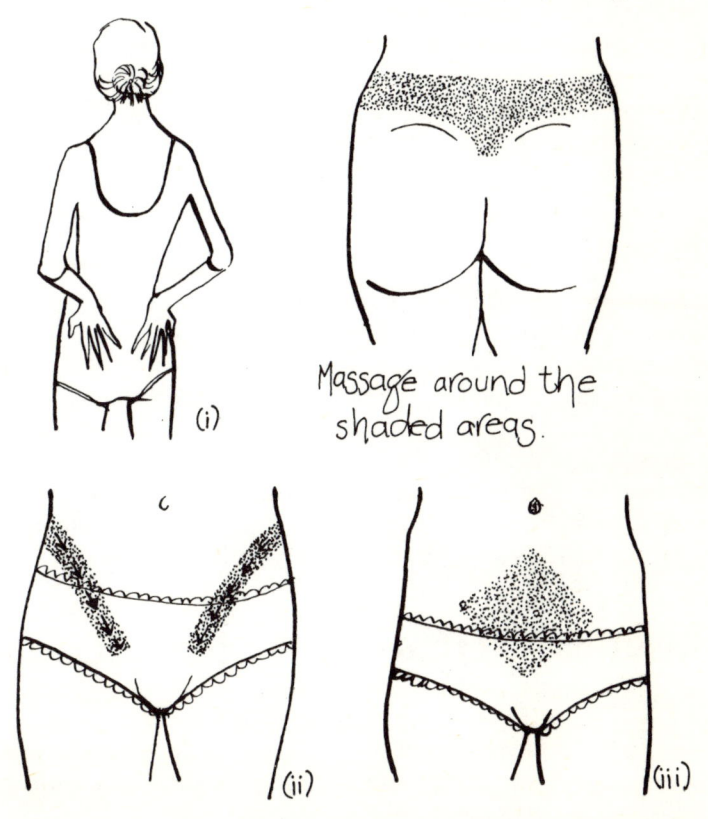

(i)

Massage around the shaded areas.

(ii)

(iii)

massage oil or deep-heating cream, available from chemists or health food shops.

Rub your lower back and buttocks, with heavy pressure over the bony part at the bottom of your spine, in the area shown in Figure i. Use your fingertips. Massage your lower tummy too. Stroke in a 'V' shape from one hipbone down to the line of your pubic hair and up to the other hipbone (Figure ii). Another method is to push firmly with your fingertips just above your pubic hair, with a circular movement (Figure iii). It is helpful to get someone to rub and massage your lower back for you.

Stop Smoking

Some women find that their period pains get better after they stop smoking. Smoking seems to increase the contractions of the womb, and nicotine reduces the blood supply to the womb; so it is worth trying to stop smoking if you can (see Chapter 7).

Painkillers

There are several effective painkillers available from chemists. Aspirin is one of the most effective. It decreases the amounts of prostaglandins and so helps relieve womb contractions. It is always best to take painkillers before the pain starts, especially if you have to keep going regardless of bad period pains. If you find painkillers useful and necessary, start taking them at the first sign of your period. But be aware that almost all drugs, even those you can buy from the chemist, can have side-effects or may be habit-forming.

Medical Treatments for Period Pains

There are several different treatments you can get from your doctor. These can be tried if you have little success in dealing with period pains on your own.

Painkillers

Conventional painkillers such as aspirin and codeine can be obtained on prescription.

Drugs to counteract the effects of prostaglandins. Several 'Prostaglandin Inhibitors' are available. These drugs are quite new and are very helpful for some women. 'Ponstan' is the most commonly prescribed.

Relief of pain usually starts about thirty to sixty minutes after taking the tablets and lasts three to four hours. It is best to take them at the first sign of your period and over the time when you usually get the worst pain. Try a low dose first as it is difficult to predict how much you will need. Increase the dose slightly each month to find the best dose for you. If your period pains are not helped by even the highest dose recommended by your doctor, then ask to try either another type of prostaglandin inhibitor or another treatment. Prostaglandin inhibitors seem to have different effects on different women and not all women respond to them.

The Pill

Doctors often prescribe the combined oral contraceptive pill to help period pains. This works by preventing ovulation. Some women find that the pill not only eases period pains when they are on it but the effects continue after stopping the pill. It may be worth trying it for a few months. It is not advised to take the pill if you are planning to get pregnant soon, since it may take a while for normal menstrual cycles and periods to return after stopping the pill.

Dilatation and Curettage (D & C)

D & C (see Chapter 4) is sometimes recommended for women who have very severe period pains and who are not helped by painkillers or hormones. It seems to help some women, but possibly only for a short time. No one is sure why it should help period pains.

6. Premenstrual Tension

Many women notice differences in how they feel, emotionally and physically, during the monthly cycle. For some, regular ups and downs are no problem. We enjoy the times of feeling good and energetic and can cope with feeling less good at other times. But some women experience more distressing changes around the time before a period. These changes are known as *premenstrual tension*.

What is Premenstrual Tension?

Even ten years ago, premenstrual tension (commonly abbreviated to *PMT*) was virtually unheard of. It is only recently that the popular label of PMT has found its way into our everyday talk, into the newspapers and magazines.

Ask a group of women how they know when their period is due. Some will shake their heads and say that their periods start unawares each month, perhaps on time, perhaps unexpectedly, but with no welcoming herald other than a predicted date on a calendar. For other women the story is quite different:

'I can tell my period is coming about eight days beforehand. First my breasts start to swell a little; they become tender. I feel slightly rounded all over and a bit bloated. About four days before my period my moods begin to change. I get short and irritable with others, the family seem to get on top of me. I want to spend more time on my own, but usually this is impossible. I get a bit low and tearful for no reason. This will go on for a few days and I'll wonder what's wrong. Then my period starts and I realise why I was feeling down, and I'll know from now on things will be OK and I'll be able to do up my skirts again.'

'A blinding headache, two days before, it never fails to come, every month.'

'I can't be bothered to do much in the few days before my period. I feel tired and want to sleep a lot.'

'In the week before my period I suddenly have all this energy. If things are going right and I'm happy I can get a lot done: it feels great. But if I'm under pressure, I get very tense, nervy, jumpy and worried: all the energy seems to go a different way.'

There are more examples of how some women feel before their periods in the list below: there are many others that women describe, too. Everyone is unique. Usually these feelings start from fourteen to two days before a period, and last until the period starts.

Examples of Common Premenstrual Changes

You may notice one or more of the following feelings before your periods:

A change in your mood

> Feeling depressed or low, irritable, worried, unable to cope, or tearful.

Feeling tired or lethargic

A change in your sleeping pattern

> You feel you need more sleep, or find it hard to get to sleep.

A change in your sexual feelings

A change in your appetite

> You feel hungrier and crave sweet foods.

A change in your ability to concentrate

> You may have more accidents.

Physical changes

> Breast tenderness; headaches; feeling swollen or bloated, especially in the tummy, ankles, fingers and eyelids; nausea;

constipation; diarrhoea; aches and pains; stomach aches; skin rashes. Women who have asthma, hay fever or epilepsy may have worse or more frequent attacks.

How to tell if you experience PMT

If you regularly feel that you change, physically or emotionally or both, in the time before your periods, and feel better once your period starts, then you probably experience PMT. The best way to tell whether these changes are occurring before your periods and not at other times, is to keep a diary for two or three months. An example of a diary is shown in Chapter 2. If the feelings you note down happen at the same time each month, two to fourteen days before your period, then the feelings are most likely PMT. Women who experience PMT can usually predict their moods and physical changes just by checking the calendar. But if the feelings you note in your diary are erratic and occur at different times, not necessarily before your periods, then your menstrual cycle is probably not the main factor involved: other things may be affecting how you feel. It is helpful to try and sort out what else is influencing your moods and physical well-being.

Who Experiences PMT?

Do all women have PMT?

If you talked to 100 women, all having regular periods, about 70 would say they notice some changes in how they feel before periods. But this does not mean that all seventy experience PMT. About ten might feel that their premenstrual feelings are quite difficult to deal with and they would like to do something about the problem: these women would say they have PMT. Two or three would find PMT really severe and troublesome, and would say it affected their lives quite a bit.

What sort of women get PMT?

There are no rules about the 'type' of women likely to experience PMT. It is certainly not confined to highly strung or 'neurotic' women. All sorts of personalities may have problems before periods, not just women with anything 'wrong' with them.

What about age?

Women of all ages notice changes before their periods. But it seems that severe PMT is more common in the 30-40 age-range than in the 'teens and early 20s, and PMT tends to get worse with age.

When might PMT start?

A few women experience premenstrual changes right from the start of their periods at puberty. More commonly, PMT starts later on, perhaps after a baby or after coming off the pill.

What about women who have had the womb removed?

Interestingly, women who have had a hysterectomy (surgical removal of the womb, leaving the ovaries intact) may continue to notice changes around the time when they would get a period. So, PMT cannot be simply due to women knowing that a period is due and expecting to feel 'premenstrual'.

Do women have PMT every month?

You may find that some months are different, depending on what you are doing and what is going on in your life. If life is smooth and easy, PMT may well not be so much of a problem as when there are many stresses and challenges to cope with.

The Effects of PMT

The most important effect of PMT is on how you feel; PMT can lead you to feel unwell and distressed for as much as two weeks out of four.

Some women also feel very worried about the effects PMT may have on other people around them, especially on small children who might not understand their mother's apparently unpredictable changes of mood. A number of women find it harder to carry out some aspects of their daily work before a period: they may be a bit clumsy; or find it difficult to concentrate; or feel a bit muddle-headed; or feel less interested in getting on with work.

What Causes PMT?

No one really knows what causes PMT, although there are several theories. It is most likely that your body, and your menstrual cycle, are partly responsible for premenstrual changes, but it is probably not the whole story. PMT is very sensitive to stress and events in your life. So your body may cause certain changes before a period, but whether these changes are felt as severe PMT or as milder ups and downs, may depend very much on life's stresses and strains. So how might your body cause your cyclical changes?

Hormones and PMT

The chances are that the hormones of the menstrual cycle are involved, since PMT is linked so closely to the time of the month. There may be a slight imbalance between oestrogens and progesterone. Perhaps your body is not making enough progesterone in the time before your period. The sudden drop in hormones in the days before a period may cause changes in how you feel. Another hormone, *prolactin*, may be involved. This is made by the pituitary gland in the brain (see Chapter 1), and causes breast tissue to produce milk when you are breast-feeding. It is also made in smaller amounts during the menstrual cycle. It is possible that too much prolactin in the second part of the menstrual cycle, before a period, may contribute to PMT, especially to breast tenderness and fluid retention.

Sensitivity to hormones

Just as people vary in how sensitive they are to alcohol and to other drugs, women may differ in how sensitive they are to their own hormones. Some women may be acutely sensitive to the changing levels of hormones during the menstrual cycle, and may experience this as PMT.

Deficiency of Vitamin B6 (Pyridoxine)

Vitamin B6 (Pyridoxine) is important in chemical processes in the body. Two of its roles may be involved in PMT. Firstly, B6 plays a part in making prolactin, such that if there is not enough B6 in your body, the pituitary gland makes too much prolactin, perhaps contributing to breast tenderness and fluid retention. Secondly, B6 may be involved in the chemistry of moods, so low levels of B6 in your body may make you feel low and depressed.

Fluid retention

Hormones control the balance of fluids and salts in the body. As a result of the change in hormones before a period, some women retain fluid, which causes the puffy, bloated feelings, and possibly tiredness, breast tenderness and headaches.

Low blood sugar

Hormones also control the amounts of sugar in the blood, necessary to supply a constant source of energy. Before a period, the levels of sugar may drop lower than usual. This causes you to feel low, tired, weak and shaky, irritable and headachy. You may also want to eat more, especially sweet foods, in order to boost up your flagging blood sugar.

What to Do about PMT

There are ways of coping with PMT. You can help yourself come to terms with and manage these regular distressing feelings. There are a number of solutions. It is a case of first understanding and analysing PMT—facing up to the problems— and then working out what is troubling you most and what you can do to help yourself.

First of all, you will need to face the problems; talk about PMT, keep a diary so that you know when to expect it, make allowances for yourself at these times, and deal with stress in your life which may exacerbate PMT. Then you must cope with specific problems such as tension, irritability and anger, fluid retention, low blood sugar, headaches and migraines and breast tenderness. Certain general remedies, e.g Vitamin B6 and Evening Primrose Oil (Efamol) may help with some or all of these.

1. Face the Problem

Talk about PMT

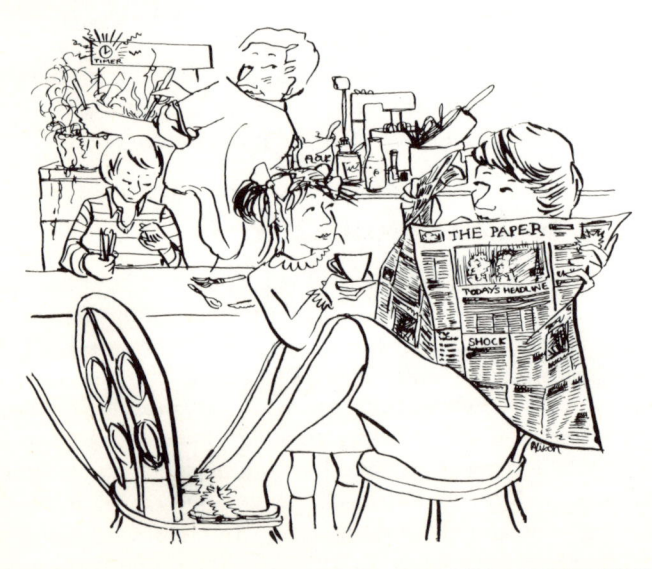

For many women it is surprising and reassuring to discover that they are not the only ones to feel as they do, and that lots of women have a problem coping with premenstrual changes. The only way to find out is for us to bring things out into the open and talk honestly about our experiences without feeling in any way 'neurotic' or abnormal. Discuss how you feel with other women, perhaps your friends or neighbours. Some Family Planning Clinics and Well Woman Clinics (see Chapter 7) organise groups for women to talk about PMT. It can be very helpful to talk things over with your family or others you live with or work with, especially if you are worried that they are affected by your premenstrual changes. Other people can help you, too. It is often unfair that so many women have to take care of all the domestic side of life as well as look after children and do a full-time job. This can all prove too much before a period. Your family and other people at home can help in many ways to relieve at least some of your domestic responsibilities.

Keep a diary

Using a diary like the one in Chapter 2, note down how you feel each day, especially anything you recognise as being connected with your periods. If you do this for a few months, you can see some pattern to your feelings. This is helpful in understanding your personal cycles of moods and physical health. It makes your changes more predictable, which is a useful step towards accepting and dealing with feelings that may be difficult at the time.

Make allowances

Make allowances for the times when you are not feeling so well. Remember that for each difficult day there will be many more good days after your period arrives. It would be nice, although not always possible, to be able to leave a few non-essential tasks undone, or get extra help, on the off-days, catching up with things later on; or to schedule important events and activities to fit with 'good' days. Do what you can to organise life to make the most of when you are not feeling premenstrual. If you are not feeling too well, think of things you can do to make yourself feel better and take time to do something positive for yourself: a long soak in a hot bath or a walk in the park, perhaps. Take up offers of activities that sound fun and out of your usual daily routine.

Dealing with stress

There is no doubt that stress plays a big part in PMT. Many women find premenstrual feelings far harder to deal with when under stress; a severe PMT sufferer can find her cyclical changes are milder and more manageable when life's pressures ease a bit. Look at stress and pressures in your life and what you can do about them. Unfortunately, the way we live can seem almost unchangeable. It is not always easy to cope with upsetting situations, difficult relationships or problems with the family and at work. But if you feel that your life is making PMT harder to cope with, try and see ways around problems.

Do not be afraid to say to yourself and to others that you are having a hard time, or that you cannot cope with things at times. We all go through periods when life is difficult. It can be a great help to talk things through and use other people for advice and support. Talking can involve a chat with a friendly neighbour; or you may prefer to talk to someone who is trained to listen and to help with problems—a counsellor or social worker. Your local Samaritans are a good starting-point—their number is in the telephone book. Your GP, Well Woman Clinic, Family Planning Clinic or Citizens' Advice Bureau may also be able to suggest people to talk to.

2. Cope with Specific Problems

Tension

Tension can be a large part of PMT: you may feel tense, worried and clenched-up. There are usually good reasons for feeling tense. Do not ignore these feelings, but try and work out what is upsetting you and what you can do about it. If you are very tense, it can be hard to start to deal with problems or worries. Tension can make you feel quite weak. Try and deal with your tension first. It helps to learn to relax, using the relaxation techniques described in Chapter 5.

Irritability and anger

A lot of women feel bad about expressing irritability and anger. They are concerned about snapping at the children, shouting, throwing things around or flying off the handle. Now that PMT is talked about so much more, anger is often lightly dismissed and put down to 'that time of the month'. But there are almost always good and valid reasons for being angry. You may be expressing things that have been annoying you all month. Try and work out what is annoying you and what you can do about it—and that includes getting angry about things. Remember, women do not have to be nice *all* the time!

Fluid retention

Fluid retention may involve feeling heavy, puffy and bloated; swollen fingers, ankles, face or eyelids; or a tightness in the skin; headaches or migraines; constipation; and possibly, sore, swollen breasts. Some women actually gain weight before their periods, whereas for others, fluid retention is due to a redistribution of body fluids, with no actual weight gain. To deal with fluid retention, you need to do three things:

Cut down salt, which makes your body retain more fluid

Drink less fluid and help your body get rid of extra fluid

Replace potassium, which is lost when you retain fluid and salt

Cut down salt

Use less salt when cooking: others eating the meal can always add more to their own food if necessary. Many foods contain a lot of salt. Some are listed below. Have a look for salt listed in the ingredients of foods you buy. Try to use less of salty foods, instead substituting foods which are low in salt: green vegetables, fresh fruit, fruit juice, rice and other grains, cereals, flour, unsalted nuts, eggs, milk, fresh fish and meat and dried fruits, for example. Fresh foods, rather than foods in tins and packets, are usually free of added salt, so buy these whenever you can.

Foods containing a lot of salt

Tinned foods: soups, fish, meat, vegetables, corned beef

Packet soups and instant meals

Smoked and cured fish and meat (kippers, sardines, ham, bacon, sausages and salami)

Cheese, butter and margarine

Stock cubes

Marmite, peanut butter, meat paste, fish paste

Soy sauce, tomato ketchup, chutney, Worcester sauce

Salad dressing, sandwich spreads

Soft drinks, tomato juice

Packeted breakfast cereals

Snacks like cheesy biscuits, crisps and salted nuts

Drink less fluid and help your body get rid of extra fluid

A lot of drinking is more habitual than due to thirst, so we take in more fluid than we actually need most of the time. Try and drink only when you are thirsty rather than because it is 'coffee time' or 'tea time'. Use small cups rather than a big mug. A piece of fruit is a nice substitute for morning or afternoon tea or coffee. Some drinks are diuretic and help the body to get rid of extra fluid. Try a range of herbal teas instead of ordinary tea. Diuretic herbal teas are listed in the Appendix. Dandelion coffee and grain coffees are also diuretic and are good substitutes for ordinary coffee; you can buy them from health food shops. Try and avoid ordinary tea and coffee if you are retaining fluid: too much caffeine, in tea and coffee, can make fluid retention worse. Some foods are also diuretic; use cucumber, artichokes, celery, aubergines or watermelon, when they are in season; prunes, figs and rhubarb also make you pass more water. You can buy mild herbal diuretic tablets from herbalists and health food shops; these help get rid of excess fluids.

Premenstrual Tension

Replace lost potassium

Oranges, bananas, tomatoes, unsalted nuts, soya beans and dried fruits are rich in potassium; eat these, rather than salty foods, before periods. Alternatively, you can buy potassium tablets from chemists and health food shops to help replace lost potassium.

Other suggestions for fluid retention

If you feel swollen and bloated, avoid large, heavy meals which seem to make things worse. Cut down on starchy foods such as cakes, biscuits, buns, puddings and sweets and fatty, fried foods; these can make you feel quite uncomfortable if you have a problem with fluid retention. Instead, have light meals.

Avoid getting constipated: constipation seems to make fluid retention worse. See Chapter 8 for remedies for constipation.

Wear comfortable clothes. If you are a bit swollen and cannot comfortably do up your tight-fitting clothes, wear loose, flowing clothes instead. Enjoy changing your image on premenstrual days.

Exercise can help fluid retention.

It is probably more helpful to deal with fluid retention before it starts rather than trying to get rid of a build-up of excess fluids and salt. If you know when you usually start to feel puffy, begin cutting down on salt and fluids, or start drinking diuretic herbal teas, before this time. Some women get black circles under their eyes before a period. This is a useful early sign of fluid retention.

A note on 'feeling fat' before a period. Many women describe premenstrual fluid retention in terms of 'feeling fat' and therefore unattractive and awful. Some talk about premenstrual weight-gain as if it were a crime for women's shape to change a bit for a few days each month. There is a lot of pressure on women always to be slim, so that women quite often feel bad about getting larger. It helps to think about what fluid retention really means to you and to how you feel about yourself; if your shape and size changes before your periods, accept it as a part of you.

Low blood sugar

Before periods, your blood sugar can fall dramatically, leaving you feeling weak, faint, irritable and low. You may crave sweet foods or want to eat more than usual. It helps to eat several small, high protein meals at regular intervals throughout the day rather than a few large meals. This means you are getting a constant supply of energy. Try and avoid going for a long time without eating and eat *before* you get too hungry. Despite craving sweet foods, sweets and chocolate can make things worse: sugar boosts up blood sugar for only a short time and makes it drop dramatically afterwards, rather than supplying long-lasting energy. Have a nutritious, sustaining snack such as a yoghurt, or cheese and fruit, or a handful of nuts, rather than a chocolate bar.

Headaches and migraines

If you are prone to headaches or migraines, you may get more, or more severe, attacks before your periods. Keep a note of when you get headaches in relation to your periods. Write down anything else associated with attacks, such as feeling faint, giddy or very hungry; stress; alcohol; or particular foods. You may be able to work out what 'triggers off' attacks. Headaches and migraines may be caused by stress, tension, fluid retention or low blood sugar, so try the remedies for these (above). Relaxation helps a great deal with headaches, especially if you can relax either before or at the first sign of an attack. Try the herbal remedies in the Appendix.

Breast tenderness

Breast tenderness may be, in part, due to fluid retention; so try the remedies for this. If your breasts are swollen and tender, wear a good-fitting stretchy bra, or a leotard. Loose dresses or shirts are more comfortable than tight jumpers. Warn your over-affectionate lover, partner or children that bear-hugs are not appreciated on certain days.

3. General Remedies

If you are troubled by a combination of physical and emotional changes before your periods, there are two remedies available which may help many aspects of PMT: Vitamin B6 and Evening Primrose Oil.

Vitamin B6 (Pyridoxine)

Vitamin B6 can help premenstrual breast tenderness, fluid retention and feeling low, tense and irritable. In low doses it is not harmful and there have been no side effects reported. B6 is sold under the name of Benadon in 20 and 50mg tablets. You can buy it from chemists. Alternatively there are various other vitamin tablets sold at health food shops, but these tend to be more expensive. The recommended dose is to start with one 50mg tablet twice a day, one at breakfast and one with the evening meal. If this does not seem to help, the dose can be increased to 150mg per day, i.e. three 50mg tablets a day or up to 200mg per day, i.e. two 50mg tablets twice a day. It is best not to take more than 200mg a day since you might get an upset stomach. Start the tablets three days before you usually begin to feel premenstrual and stop on the second or third day of your period, or whenever your discomfort usually eases.

It is usually necessary to experiment to find out the best dosage for you: some women need a higher dose than others. Try one dose for two cycles. If it does not help, then increase the dose for the next two cycles; continue increasing the dose, if necessary, up to the maximum of 200mg per day. Not all women find B6 helpful, even at the highest dose, so you may need to try something else. But for some women B6 takes a couple of months to work, so it is worth persevering even if there are no dramatic changes in the first cycle. If it is helping, continue B6 for three to four months, then stop for a month to see if the PMT returns. Sometimes a few months on the vitamin is enough to help in the long term. If PMT returns when you stop, then repeat B6 for another three or four cycles, again stopping to see if you no longer need to take it.

Recently, it has been suggested that the effects of B6 may be improved by taking additional magnesium. If you find B6 is not helping PMT, try improving your dietary intake of magnesium, by eating more wholegrains, green leafy vegetables, nuts, seeds, or brewers yeast; or take magnesium supplements, available from health food shops, of 200-300 mg per day whilst taking B6.

Evening primrose oil (Efamol)

The oil from the evening primrose, made under the name of 'Efamol', is a newly-available remedy for PMT. You buy it from health food shops and chemists. The oil contains a fatty acid, gamma linoleic acid, which is important for many of the body's functions, including the menstrual cycle. It is claimed that gamma linoleic acid helps correct imbalances in the body which may contribute to PMT and also, possibly, to heavy periods. Efamol is still being tested to see how effective it is. Quite a few women find it helps premenstrual headaches, fluid retention, breast tenderness, breast pains, aching joints, irritability, depression and anxiety. Some women find it makes their periods lighter. Some women who have not been helped by vitamin B6 have had more success with Efamol, so it may be worth a try.

Efamol products are available from health food shops and chemists. You take either Efamol 250 or Efamol 500, with an extra vitamin supplement Efavite; alternatively, Efamol PMP combines Efamol with vitamins. Take it as directed on the packet. It may be necessary to take Efamol every day for two months, then for only part of the menstrual cycle, from three days before you expect PMT to start until your period. Efamol seems to have few side-effects; occasionally women taking it get facial spots or feel a bit depressed. Efamol is quite expensive, although it may become available on prescription from a doctor.

Self-help remedies may be very effective in coming to terms with and dealing with PMT. However, if nothing seems to help or you feel that things are too difficult to cope with on your own, there are treatments available from the doctor. You may need drugs to help you for a while, perhaps whilst you work out ways of dealing with PMT in the long term.

Help from the Doctor

Your doctor can prescribe a number of treatments. Usually, by a process of trial and error, you can find a suitable drug to help you.

When you go to your doctor it is useful to take a menstrual diary, showing the changes that are worrying you and when they occur in relation to your periods. Keep a diary when you are taking treatments, too, so you can see if there is any change in the premenstrual feelings.

Progesterone

The hormone progesterone seems to help some women. It is taken either as *natural progesterone* or in a synthetic (artificial) form called *Progestogen*.

Natural progesterone was widely used before the newer synthetic hormones became available. You cannot take it as tablets, by mouth; it must be taken either as injections or as pessaries put in the vagina or rectum. You start the treatment five days before you usually start to feel 'premenstrual' and continue it until your period starts. The dose must be carefully worked out to suit each individual, since some women need more progesterone than others. Working out the right dose for you can take a while. Natural progesterone can be very helpful to some women, although some find it makes little or no difference to PMT and others feel worse whilst taking progesterone. There may be some side-effects, such as the inconvenience or discomfort of daily injections; unpleasant or messy leakage from vaginal or rectal pessaries; pessaries may make you more prone to vaginal infections such as thrush; and some women get breast tenderness or fluid retention, or feel depressed whilst taking progesterone.

Progestogens (synthetic progesterones). Dydrogesterone, called Duphaston, is the most widely used progestogen. About 70 per cent of women who take it feel that it helps PMT, especially with fluid retention and sometimes with depression, tension and irritability. It is not usually useful for breast tenderness. You take Duphaston as 10mg tablets twice a day, starting about twelve days after a period and continuing until two days before you expect your next period. If Duphaston does not help at first, alter when you take it: for example, take the tablets every day; or start earlier in your cycle, perhaps five days after your period starts. You may need a higher dose, perhaps up to 15 to 20mg twice a day.

Not many women notice side-effects on the lower doses of Duphaston, although it occasionally causes breast tenderness, mild nausea, headaches or migraines, or it can make varicose veins worse. There may be more risks of side-effects if you take higher doses. It is impossible to predict Duphaston's effects on your periods; while taking the hormone, some women have irregular periods, some have more regular periods and others notice no change. You will need to try Duphaston for at least three months to see whether it helps PMT. Sometimes a combination of Duphaston and Vitamin B6 can help if B6 alone or Duphaston alone makes little or no difference.

The oral contraceptive pill

It may be worth trying the combined oral contraceptive pill for a few months to see if it helps. The pill has different effects on different women. Some find it very helpful. A short time on the pill may be enough to alleviate PMT; after taking the pill for a few months, some women find PMT does not reappear when they stop taking it. However, some women find it makes no difference; and a number of women cannot tolerate the pill and feel unwell all the time whilst taking it.

Diuretics

Your doctor can prescribe diuretic tablets to help you deal with fluid retention. Diuretics will not necessarily affect your moods or depression, or breast tenderness. Diuretics will make you pass water more frequently and may give you a dry mouth. If you use diuretics for a long time, there may be a risk of running low on potassium. This can be remedied either by increasing potassium-rich foods in your diet (see Chapter 8) or by taking additional potassium, prescribed by the doctor.

Other Treatments from the Doctor

Progesterone, the pill and diuretics are the most commonly prescribed treatments. Your doctor may also recommend and prescribe Vitamin B6 or Efamol. One or a combination of these drugs usually helps most women. But if they do not help and your PMT is persistent and severe, there are other drugs available. Your doctor may recommend one of these.

Occasionally a drug called *Spironolactone* is prescribed for severe and troublesome fluid retention. It alters the systems in your body involved in regulating fluids and salt. Little is known about its side-effects or long-term effects.

Bromocriptine is a drug that reduces the amounts of prolactin in the body. Your doctor may test your prolactin levels, using a blood test. High prolactin may cause severe breast tenderness and possibly fluid retention. Bromocriptine can cause side-effects, such as nausea during the first ten to fourteen days you take it; lowering of blood pressure; dizziness and visual disturbances.

Although *tranquillisers* and *antidepressants* are sometimes prescribed for PMT, they are not often helpful. If PMT only affects you for part of the time and you feel fine otherwise, it may not be appropriate to take drugs that affect your moods all the time. The drugs can make you feel tired and lethargic, especially when you first start to take them. However, if you are very worried or agitated or depressed, tranquillisers or antidepressants can be very useful whilst you sort out the causes of feeling low.

PMT Clinics

Special clinics to help with PMT have been set up, usually attached to the gynaecology department of a hospital. You can attend these as an out-patient. Your GP may refer you to a clinic if there is one in your area.

Department of Gynaecology, St Thomas's Hospital, Lambeth Palace Road, London SE1 7EH

PMT Clinic, Elizabeth Garrett Anderson Hospital, 144 Euston Road, London NW1 2AP 01-387 2501

Periods

Queenswood Unit, Middlewood Hospital, PO Box 134, Sheffield S6 1TP 0742 349491 ext. 286

Family Planning Association, 17 North Church Street, Sheffield S1 2DH 0742 21191

Department of Obstetrics and Gynaecology, City Hospital, Hucknall Road, Nottingham NG5 1PB 0602 608111

Dr J. Bancroft, Gynaecology Out-Patients Department, Royal Infirmary, Lauriston Place, Edinburgh 031-229 2477

The Pre-Menstrual Syndrome Clinic, Department of Obstetrics and Gynaecology, The Royal Free Hospital, Pond Street, Hampstead, London NW3 2QG 01-794 0500 Ext. 3836

PMS Clinic, Department of Obstetrics and Gynaecology, St George's Hospital, Blackshaw Road, London SW17 0QT 01-627 1255

PMS Clinic, MRC Mineral Metabolism Unit, General Infirmary, Great George Street, Leeds LS1 3EX 0532 432799

PMS Clinic, Department of Obstetrics and Gynaecology, Stobhill Hospital, Glasgow G21 3UW 041-558 0111

Dr Ann Parker, Family Planning Clinic, Nevill Hall Hospital, Abergavenny (Letters only)

PMS Clinic, Department of Psychological Medicine, Whitchurch Hospital, Cardiff 0222 62191

Cardiff Well Woman Advisory Centre, 15 Richmond Crescent, Cardiff CF2 3TJ

The Well Woman Centre of Marie Stopes House, London, runs a clinic on Saturday mornings, to which you can refer yourself, without a GP referral. The clinic is a private charity so a low fee is charged. Telephone for an appointment: 01-388 0662 or 01-388 2585. The address is: Marie Stopes House, The Well Woman Centre, 108 Whitfield Street, London W1P 6BE.

7. Help For Period Problems

There are some problems with periods that are best diagnosed and treated by a qualified medical practitioner. It is good to seek advice if you feel that something is wrong, if you are not quite sure of the causes and if you do not know how to help yourself. Self-help may not always be easy. Sometimes, it is hard to know where to begin to make changes for better health, or nothing really seems to work. There are many trained practitioners available to help with period problems.

Help from the Doctor

Your doctor is the most obvious and easily-available source of help. When you see your doctor, tell her all your symptoms and details of when they started and what they are connected with. Tell her the dates of your periods and show her your menstrual diary (see Chapter 2). It helps to note down what you want to say before your appointment, so you can make the best use of the short time available with your GP. You may like to talk things over with a friend or relative beforehand, or perhaps ask someone to come with you. Make sure you fully understand what the doctor thinks is wrong and the treatment. Your doctor can refer you to a specialist, usually a gynaecologist, for further diagnosis, tests and treatment. You are always entitled to another medical opinion, especially for major problems.

You may feel that you do not want to discuss your period problems with your doctor, or she may not be helpful. See another doctor, rather than not going to the doctor or remaining dissatisfied with your treatment. Ask around for names of good doctors. Your Community Health Council (their number is in the telephone book) may be able to recommend doctors who are especially helpful for period problems. You may prefer to see a woman doctor. The Family Practitioner Committee have lists of doctors. You can see the list at libraries, main post offices and Citizens' Advice Bureaux. If you want to change your doctor, the procedure is explained on your medical card. The easiest way is to send your card to the Family Practitioner Committee, explaining that you wish to leave your present doctor and register with another. You do not necessarily have to get your doctor's consent to leave the the practice.

Doctors at Family Planning Clinics and Brook Advisory Centres are often helpful and sympathetic about period problems. You can attend these clinics without a referral from your doctor. Telephone and ask for an appointment. The numbers are in the telephone book. For more information on how to get the best from your doctor, see the books listed at the end.

Well Woman Clinics

These are clinics to help women achieve and maintain good health rather than dealing with illnesses. You can get advice on general health, menstrual and menopausal problems, contraception, pregnancy and childbirth, thrush, cystitis, eating problems, social and emotional difficulties and other aspects of health. Clinics test for cervical and breast cancers and teach self-examination. To find out whether there is a Well Woman Clinic in your area, get in touch with your Family Practitioner Committee, District Health Authority or Community Health Council. Their numbers are in the telephone book.

Alternative Medicine

Various branches of alternative medicine offer help for period problems. Alternative medicine is not usually available on the National Health Service. This means that you have to pay for consultation and treatment. However, some practitioners have a sliding scale of charges, so you pay what you can afford, according to your income.

Most alternative health practitioners view symptoms, such as period problems, in terms of the whole body being unhealthy or unbalanced in some way. Advice and treatment is concerned with your lifestyle and general health. So as well as using specific techniques of treatment, practitioners will give you advice on exercise, relaxation, nutrition and your emotional wellbeing and lifestyle.

If you want to consult one of the practitioners of alternative medicine, write to the address given below each section, sending a large stamped, self-addressed envelope for a list of local registered practitioners.

Homeopathy

Homeopaths use tiny amounts of naturally-occurring substances from plants and animals, which somehow stimulate the body's system of defence against illness and so restore health. Some homeopathic doctors work under the National Health Service and there are NHS homeopathic hospitals, so you can get free treatment. Any GP can write prescriptions for homeopathic remedies. You can also buy homeopathic remedies from chemists and health food shops.

Contact The British Homeopathic Association, 27A Devonshire Street, London W1N 1RJ 01-935 2163.

Herbalism

Herbalism was the main system of medicine until chemical drugs became widely used. Herbalists use plants with medicinal value to prevent and cure disease and to restore the body's healthy balance. Herbalists make up their own remedies, tailor-made for each patient. The remedies are in very small doses and, unlike many modern drugs, side-effects are rare.

Contact The National Institute of Medical Herbalists, PO Box 3, Winchester SO22 6RB 0962 68776.

Naturopathy

Naturopaths believe that the body is able to make itself healthy by using its own healing forces. They aim to discover and remove whatever is preventing the healing processes and causing disease, such as faulty nutrition, breathing, bowel or bladder functions, structural or postural faults or emotional problems. Naturopaths work principally on nutrition and diet.

Contact The British Naturopathic and Osteopathic Association, 6 Netherhall Gardens, London NW3 5RR 01-435 8728.

Osteopathy

Osteopaths believe that many health problems are due to the structure of the body, particularly the bones, joints and muscles, not working properly. The treatment involves manipulation of the body. Osteopathy also rebalances the nervous system regulating basic functions, including the hormones and the menstrual cycle.

Contact The British Osteopathic Association, 8-10 Boston Place, London NW1 6QH 01-262 5250.

Chiropractic

Chiropractors specialise in backs and spines, and believe that spinal problems affect the nervous system. Since the nervous system affects all parts of the body, skilful manipulations of the spine can remedy all sorts of problems, not just those directly concerned with the back. Chiropractic adjustments of the pelvis and lower back may help the reproductive system and remedy period problems.

Contact The British Chiropractors' Association, 5 First Avenue, Chelmsford, Essex CM1 1RX 0245 358487.

Acupuncture

Acupuncture is part of the Chinese system of medicine. It is a painful-sounding but painless technique of inserting needles into various points on the body, corresponding to different organs and systems, to 'unblock' channels of energy and so restore healthy functioning.

Contact The British Acupuncture Association and Register, 34 Alderney Street, London SW1V 4EU 01-834 3353 or 01-834 1012.

Self-Help Groups

Many women find it a great help to talk things through with other women with similar problems. You can share your concerns, swap remedies and support each other whilst making changes to get well. To find out about self-help groups in your area, ask your local Family Planning Clinic or Well Woman Clinic. Several organisations can put you in touch with local groups: The Women's Therapy Centre; The Women's Health Information Centre; Help for Health; and WIRES. Their addresses are at the end of the book. Self-help groups have been set up by women suffering from endometriosis and premenstrual tension, and by women after a hysterectomy. Addresses of these groups are also at the end.

8. Helping Yourself With Period Problems

If you have a problem with your periods, whether heavy periods, painful periods, no periods or premenstrual tension, your general health may not be as good as it could be, and period problems may be a symptom of this. Rather than just dealing with the symptoms, it is worth having a look at all aspects of your health, not just your periods. General health means paying attention to what you eat; exercise; sleep, rest and relaxation. Many women spend so much time looking after others' health that they forget themselves in small but important ways. Women are finding that improving their general health, perhaps through changing their diet, taking more exercise, learning yoga or learning to relax, has made a big difference to seemingly impossible period problems.

Diet and Nutrition

Women need a good balanced diet. It is easy to overlook your own dietary needs and not get enough of the right food, especially if you shop and cook for the rest of the household.

Many tinned, packaged and processed foods have lost a lot of their nutritional value; they are low on vitamins and minerals and instead are loaded with artificial preservatives and chemicals. We tend to eat too much fat, especially animal fat; too much sugar and salt; too few vegetables and not enough fibre. Try eating fresh foods rather than foods from tins or packets: fresh fruit and vegetables, for example. Eat wholegrain products: wholemeal bread rather than white bread; use wholemeal flour in baking; brown rice rather than white; wholegrain cereals, such as oats or muesli, rather than packeted breakfast cereals. Wholefood and health food shops and many supermarkets stock grains, wholemeal flour and bread, and cereals. Try to eat less sugar. Fresh and dried fruit and honey are just as satisfying for a sweet tooth. Vegetarians

Helping Yourself

seem to get fewer period problems than meat eaters. It may help to cut down on meat. Substitute vegetable proteins from beans and lentils, nuts and seeds, fish, eggs, low-fat cheeses, yoghurt, tofu and soya bean products such as TVP. It is good to cut down on fat in your diet. It is very easy to run low on essential vitamins and minerals. Have a look at this table to check that your daily diet includes some of the foods for each vitamin and mineral.

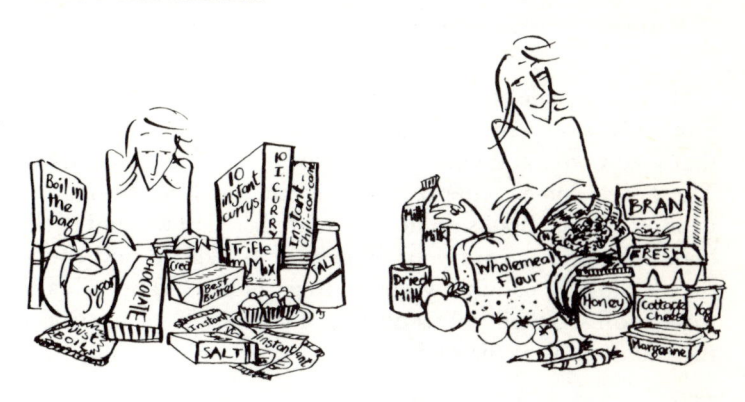

Vitamins and Minerals important for good health

1. Vitamins	Good Sources
A	Liver; oily fish such as herrings, sardines, fish-liver oils; butter; margarine; eggs; milk; carrots; spinach; peaches; apricots
B1 (Thiamin)	Wholemeal flour and bread; wheatgerm; cereals such as oats, muesli; brown rice; brewers yeast; milk; nuts; meat; potatoes
B2 (Riboflavin)	Liver; eggs; milk; cereals; brewers yeast
Niacin	Meat; fish; wholemeal flour and bread; wheatgerm; brewers yeast; cereals
Folic Acid	Liver; green vegetables; cereals; eggs; brown rice
B6 (Pyridoxine)	Meat; fish; wholemeal flour and bread; cereals; nuts; beans; peas; bananas
B12	Liver; fish; milk; eggs
C	Fresh fruit and vegetables
D	Liver; oily fish such as herrings, sardines; fish-liver oils; butter; margarine; eggs; cheese

Periods

E	Wholemeal flour and bread; wheatgerm; vegetable oils; eggs; milk; green vegetables
2. Minerals	Good Sources
Calcium	Cheese; milk; eggs; flour and bread
Iron	Liver; meat; eggs; flour and bread; wheatgerm; green vegetables; potatoes; dried fruit; peanuts; molasses
Potassium	Fresh and dried fruit such as oranges, bananas, figs, prunes; vegetables; wholemeal flour and bread; cereals
Magnesium	Green vegetables; wholemeal flour and bread; grains such as millet; brewers yeast

If you decide to alter your diet, make the changes gradually, slowly introducing new foods or ways of cooking so that your body, and your family, can get used to the changes. These are some general ideas about good nutrition and healthy eating. Books on nutrition are listed at the end of the book. Get some from your library or bookshop and spend time thinking about your eating habits. The Health Education Council will send you information on nutrition: their address is at the end.

Avoid getting constipated. Eat lots of fresh fruit, and vegetables high in fibre, such as cabbage, carrots and potatoes. Prunes, figs and rhubarb help avoid constipation. Wholemeal bread and wholegrain products supply extra fibre. Try adding extra bran to your diet. Start with two teaspoons a day, sprinkled on cereal, yoghurt or stewed fruit, and gradually increase to two tablespoons daily. Drinking extra water can help constipation, although not if you have problems with fluid retention. Drink an extra glass of water before meals, and avoid getting dehydrated.

Some other remedies for occasional constipation:

Soak one teaspoon of linseeds (available from health food shops) in one cup of boiling water for two hours, then drink the liquid and eat the seeds.

Try elderflower tea (see Appendix for making herbal teas).

Try a honey-cider vinegar drink first thing in the morning: put one teaspoon of honey and half a teaspoon of cider vinegar in a cup of boiling water.

Food Allergies

We all know someone who cannot live with cats, sneezes at household dust or gets hay fever. Most people can mention one food which they avoid, knowing it causes sickness or a rash. Recently a lot of common foods have been linked to a variety of health problems, including period problems. By detecting certain culprits in their diets and avoiding these foods, some women find their periods much easier to cope with. If you would like more details about food allergies, there are some books in the 'Further Reading' list, or contact 'Action Against Allergy': their address is at the end.

Coffee and Tea

Caffeine, found in coffee and tea, has recently been linked with period problems. It might help to cut down on or give up caffeine. Try some substitutes for tea and coffee, such as 'decaffeinated' coffee and grain coffee; herbal teas; fruit juice and mineral waters. Use your ingenuity and try a variety of drinks. Apart from being healthier you may find it more interesting and enjoyable than endless cups of the same ordinary tea and coffee.

Smoking and Alcohol

Smoking and drinking may not help with period problems, although it is, of course, hard to tell whether they cause problems, or whether we use cigarettes and alcohol to cope with stresses and feeling unwell. It has been found that many women with period problems also smoke and drink, so it is worth trying to cut down or give up to see if it helps. The Health Education Council (address at the end) can send information.

Exercise

Exercise is especially important for women to keep our reproductive systems in order, as well as being good for our general health, fitness and well-being. Find something you enjoy doing and will do, and add exercise to your daily routine. Take or make time for walking, jogging, swimming, tennis, badminton, keep-fit or whatever. There are lots of classes: your local library or Citizens' Advice Bureau can provide details. The Health Education Council (address at the end) will send information on exercise. If you are disabled, it may not be so easy to exercise. There are classes, such as yoga, swimming, keep fit and 'Look After Yourself' for disabled people. Contact the Health Education Council, Disabled Living Foundation or Liberation Network for information (addresses at the end).

Yoga

Yoga is becoming a very popular form of exercise and relaxation. Many women are finding great relief from persistent period problems through regular practice of yoga. Many of the exercises are especially good for women; they make the hormonal systems, reproductive systems and pelvic area healthy and balanced. It is best to learn yoga in a class, if possible, so you learn to do the exercises correctly. Classes are also more enjoyable than learning on your own. Find out about local classes from your library or community education centre or Citizens' Advice Bureau. There are some books on yoga listed in 'Further Reading'.

Sleep and Relaxation

Getting enough sleep is important for general health, although it is not always easy for women with young children to see to their own needs for sleep. You may find that you need different amounts of sleep at different times; perhaps more, perhaps less, before your periods. If you need more sleep, try to get to bed earlier, avoid planning late-night activities, and if possible sleep on longer in the morning. If you cannot get to sleep, it may be that your body does not need so much sleep. It is better to get up and do things or read until you do feel sleepy, rather than trying to get to sleep. Or try some remedies for insomnia:

Don't eat a big meal before bedtime.

Avoid caffeine: coffee and tea wake you up.

Drink chamomile tea or lime-flower tea or a hot milky drink before bed.

Have a warm bath, with lavender or rosemary oil in the water.

Listen to relaxing music, or read non-exciting books, before bedtime.

Try relaxation exercises (see Chapter 5).

Relaxation helps your general health. If you are generally very tense, try and take time to relax and learn the relaxation techniques in Chapter 5. Some women find meditation very useful in coping with tension. Here is a simple meditation exercise:

Sit comfortably in a quiet place, close your eyes and become aware of your breathing. Simply feel your breath going in and out. Count each time you breathe out, from one up to ten. When you become distracted by other thoughts, gently return your mind to your breath and to counting the out breaths. It is good to practise meditation regularly, for a few minutes each day.

Taking care of your health does not just mean waiting until you feel unwell and then doing something to help; it means getting into good habits so that doing all you can to feel well and prevent period problems becomes part of your daily life. So rather than just eating well or taking exercise around period-times, make sure you help yourself be well all the time.

Appendix

Herbs for Period Problems

There are numerous traditional remedies based on herbs, used by our great-grandmothers and their great-grandmothers to help period problems. As we have now come to use modern drugs, herbal remedies have been forgotten. But many women find them to be gentle, safe and effective alternatives to conventional medications. You can buy herbs from herbalists or from health food shops. Some herbal remedies are in tablet form. Alternatively, you can buy the herbs and take them as a herbal tea. You usually buy herbs in one or two ounce packets, or as teabags.

To make herbal tea: put half an ounce of the herb into a small teapot (not an aluminium pot). Pour on one large tea-cup of boiling water and leave to brew for 10-15 minutes. If you buy teabags, soak one bag in a cup of boiling water for 10 minutes. Strain the tea and drink it whilst it is hot. Add a little honey or lemon to taste, although many herb teas are delicious alone.

The table shows herbs recommended for period problems. Try out one or a few of the herbs to see which ones work for you.

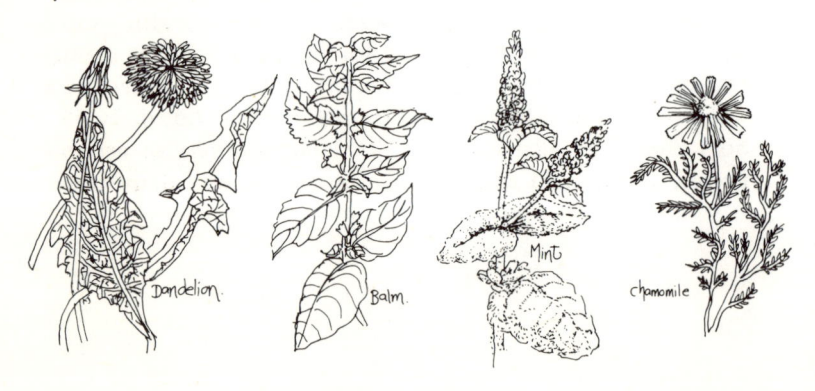

Appendix

Problem	Herbal Teas	When to take the tea
Painful periods	Raspberry leaf; Chamomile; Lemon Balm; Motherwort; White Deadnettle; Yarrow; Pasque Flower; Angelica; Rosemary; Red Clover; Mint; Parsley; Pennyroyal; Marjoram. Chamomile remedy: Brew ½ oz chamomile in 1pt boiling water for ten minutes. Strain and add to ½ oz crampbark and a pinch of powdered ginger. Simmer for ten minutes.	One cup every two hours for severe pain or one cup three times a day before and during a period.
Premenstrual depression	Lemon Balm; Chamomile; Rosemary; Sage; Borage; Fennel.	One cup, three times a day when PMT starts
Premenstrual tension and irritability	Lemon Balm; Chamomile; Hops; Lime-flowers.	One cup, three times a day when PMT starts
Premenstrual tiredness	Basil; Borage; Fennel.	One cup, three times a day when PMT starts
Premenstrual fluid retention: diuretic herbs	Dandelion leaf; Chamomile; Lemon Balm; Parsley; Mint; Pennyroyal; Marjoram; Blackcurrant; Buchu; Hibiscus; Couch Grass; Horsetail; Cornsilk; Juniper	One cup, three times a day when PMT starts
Headaches	Motherwort; Chamomile; Feverfew; Lavender; Lime-flowers; Lemon Balm; Hops; Skullcap; Peppermint; Rosemary	One cup, three times a day when PMT starts

Periods

Yoga Exercises to help with Period Problems

Here is a series of yoga exercises or 'poses' which may help with period problems. All these poses are good for the pelvic area and reproductive systems and stimulate the kidneys, keeping everything functioning properly. Ideally, you should try and practise the poses every day, or as often as you can. The poses are also good for relieving period pains if you do them when your period starts. The beauty of yoga is that you can do it almost anywhere: whilst watching television, chatting to a friend or sitting on the floor with the children.

Wear loose clothes, not tight jeans or constricting waistbands. Take off your shoes. For some of the poses you will need a blanket or pile of magazines to sit on, and a belt.

1. Hero pose (Virasana)

Start this sequence of yoga poses by sitting in Hero pose. Sit on the floor on your heels, in a kneeling position. Then move your feet apart, with your feet facing directly back, and sit

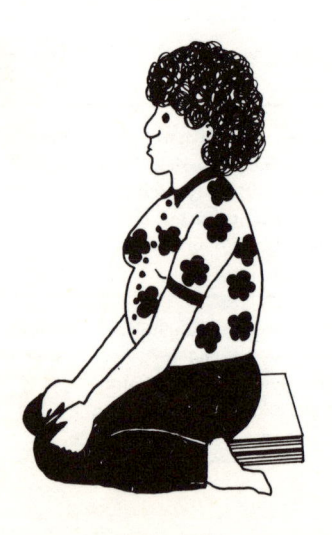

Appendix

down with your bottom on the floor between your feet. If this is not possible, and your feet or ankles hurt, then sit on a folded blanket or pile of magazines between your feet. Your feet should be close to your thighs, with the tops of your feet on the ground, and your knees should be together. Put your hands on your knees and sit upright with a straight back and relaxed shoulders. Relax your abdomen and breathe softly and gently.

Start by sitting in Hero pose for half a minute. Each time you practise, increase the time, building up to three minutes. Once you are used to the pose, it becomes a very comfortable way to sit.

2. Cobbler's pose (Baddha Konasana)

From Hero pose, move to sit in Cobbler's pose. Draw back your heels in close to your body, pressing the soles of your feet together, bending your knees, and let your knees drop down. Rest your hands behind you on the floor and try to sit up very straight. If you cannot sit up and tend to roll backwards on to the base of your spine, sit on a rolled up blanket or pile of

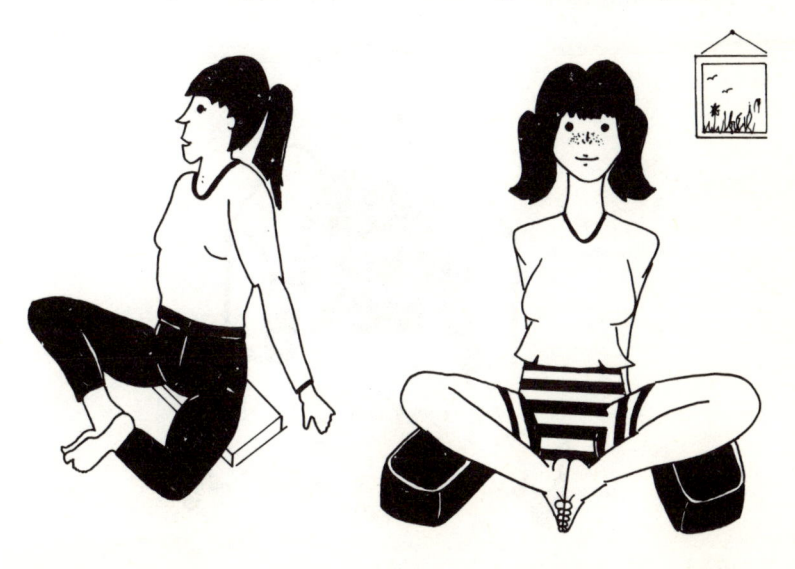

Periods

magazines (i), or sit with your back against an armchair or wall. Stretch your back up while you relax in your thighs and groin, pressing your heels together. If your thighs are high in the air, put a cushion under them to support your legs (ii). This helps you to relax across the groin.

Start by sitting in Cobbler's pose for one minute, gradually increasing to three to five minutes; keep your breathing slow and steady, concentrating on relaxing your pelvic area. As you sit in Cobbler's pose you can also practise the Pelvic Rock (see Chapter 5). Try and tilt your pelvis backwards as though trying to push the very base of your spine out from behind you. Hold for a few seconds; then tilt your pelvis the other way, tucking the base of your spine underneath you. Hold for a few seconds. Do this five to ten times.

3. *Seated angle pose (Upavistha Konasana)*

From Cobbler's pose, straighten your legs and stretch them out in front of you; then spread your legs wide apart, if necessary resting your hands on the floor behind you for support. If you

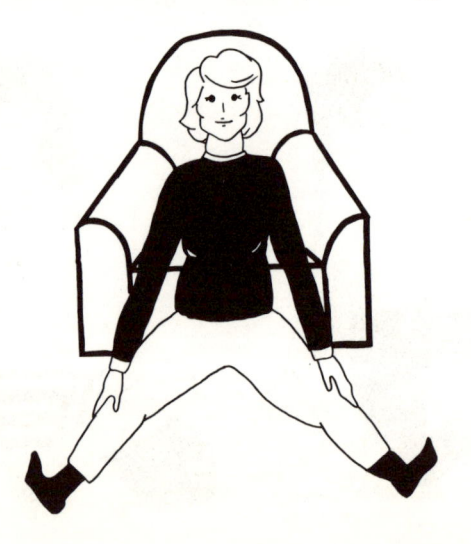

Appendix

find it hard to sit up straight, sit on your blanket or magazines or with your back supported. Keep your legs very straight, tightening your knees. Stretch your back up and try and push your body forward slightly. Feel your groin and inner thighs stretching and try and relax here. Sit like this for thirty seconds; then try to take your legs a bit further apart to increase the stretch. You can also try pressing your feet against a wall to stretch your thighs and groin more.

Start by sitting in Seated Angle pose for thirty seconds, increasing to three to five minutes. You can also do the Pelvic Rock, as for Cobbler's pose.

4. Staff pose (Dandasana)

Sit with your legs straight out in front of you, with your back upright, and rest your fingertips on the floor by your hips for balance. Sit up as straight as you can: you may need to sit on a blanket or magazines; or if you find it hard to sit with your legs together, take your feet one foot apart. Make your back as long as possible, not letting it collapse outwards so that you hunch over. It sounds like an easy exercise, but in fact it is

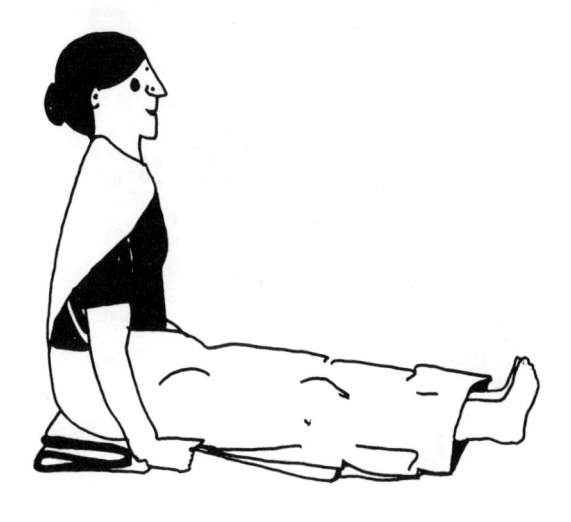

Periods

quite difficult to sit up straight. Try to sit forward on your buttock bones, pushing your bottom out behind you, as in the Pelvic Rock.

Sit for ten seconds, gradually building up to one to five minutes.

5. Forward bend (Paschimottanasana)

From Staff pose, begin to bend forward from your hips. Keep your back long and stretched and move your waist area forward, making your back hollow and convex, pushing down on the floor with your hands. Loop a belt around your feet and pull on it to stretch forward more, so your ribs move forward. Relax your stomach and feel your back and front stretching. Don't hunch your shoulders, but keep your chest open. Start by sitting like this for ten seconds, increasing to one to three minutes.

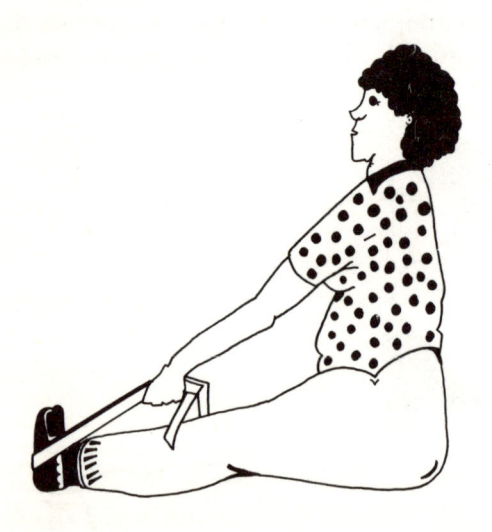

Further Reading

The Biology of Periods

The Menstrual Cycle — E. W. Wilson and P. Rennie (Lloyd-Luke, 1976)

The Cycling Female. Her Menstrual Rhythm — A. Lein (W. H. Freeman, 1979)

Female Cycles — P. Weideger (The Women's Press, 1978)

Managing Periods

Have You Started Yet? — R. Thomson (Piccolo, 1980)

Disabled Eve: Aids in Menstruation — B. P. McCarthy (Disabled Living Foundation, 1981)

Periods, Period Problems, Pains and PMT

Why Suffer? Periods and their Problems — L. Birke and K. Gardner (Virago, 1982)

Lifting the Curse. How to relieve painful periods — B. Kingston (Sheldon Press, 1984)

PMT: The Unrecognised Illness — J. Lever (New English Library, 1980)

The Wise Wound — P. Shuttle and P. Redgrove (Penguin, 1980)

No More Menstrual Cramps — P. Wise-Budoff (Angus and Robertson, 1984)

Periods

Periods without Pain	E. Wright (Star Books, 1979)
Premenstrual Tension	M. G. Brush (Pan, 1984)
Once a Month	K. Dalton (Fontana, 1984)
Premenstrual Syndrome and Progesterone Therapy	K. Dalton (Heinemann, Second Edition, 1984)
Pre-Menstrual Syndrome	C. Shreeve (Thorsons, 1983)

Books on Women's Health

Our Bodies, Ourselves	A. Phillips and J. Rakusen (Penguin, Second Edition, 1985)
From Woman to Woman	L. Lanson (Penguin, 1983)
The Good Health Guide for Women	C. W. Cooke & S. Dworkin (Hamlyn, 1981)
Below the Belt: A Guide to Gynaecological Problems	V. Welburn (W.H. Allen, 1982)
Caring for Women's Health	J. Jenkins (Search Press, 1985)
Menopause: A Positive Approach	R. Reitz (Unwin, 1981)
Menopause	J. Rakusen (Health Education Council, 1985)
Hysterectomy	L. Dennerstein (Oxford University Press, 1982)
Fat is a Feminist Issue	S. Orbach (Hamlyn, 1979)
The Pill	J. Guillebaud (Oxford University Press, 1984)

Books on General Health, Nutrition and Exercise

The Health and Fitness Handbook: A Family Guide	M. Polunin (Sphere Books, 1983)
The Right Way to Eat	M. Polunin (J. M. Dent, 1984)

Laurel's Kitchen: A Handbook for Vegetarian Cookery and Nutrition	L. Robertson (Routledge and Kegan Paul, 1979)
Quit Smoking	M. Stoppard (Ariel Books, 1982)
The Ladykillers. Why Smoking is a Feminist Issue	B. Jacobson (Pluto, 2nd Edition, 1985)
Eating and Allergy	R. Eagle (Futura, 1979)
Overcoming Food Allergies	G. H. Davies (Ashgrove Press, 1985)

Yoga

The Concise Light on Yoga	B.K.S. Iyengar (Unwin, 1980)
Tackle Yoga	S. Hoare (Stanley Paul, 1982)

Herbs

The Home Herbal	B. Griggs (Pan, 1983)

Alternative Medicines

Alternative Medicine: A Guide to Natural Therapies	A. Stanway (Penguin, 1982)
The Encyclopaedia of Alternative Medicine and Self Help	M. Hulke (Rider, 1978)

Women and Doctors

Talking to Your Doctor	C. Faulder (Virago, 1978)
Making the Most of your Doctor	J. King, D. Pendleton and P. Tate (Thames T.V., 1985)

Useful Addresses and Organisations

The Health Education Council,
78 New Oxford Street,
London WC1A 1AH
(or contact your local health education unit; the address can be found in the telephone directory)

Publishes leaflets on general health, nutrition, alcohol and women's health.

Scottish Health Education Group, Woodburn House, Canaan Lane,
Edinburgh EH10 4SG
031-447 8044

Publishes leaflets on general health, nutrition, alcohol and women's health.

Help for Health,
Wessex Regional Library Unit,
South Academic Block,
Southampton General Hospital,
Southampton SO9 4XY
0703 777222, ext. 3753

Supplies addresses of helpful organisations and details about books and leaflets on women's health

Women's Health Information Centre, 52 Featherstone Street, London EC1

Provides information on women's health and addresses of local groups and organisations.

Women's Health Concern,
Ground Floor Flat,
17 Earls Terrace,
London W8 6LP
01-602 6669

Publishes booklets on period problems and women's health.

WIRES,
(Women's Information, Referral and Enquiry Service)
PO Box 20, Oxford
0865 240991

An information centre, giving details of women's groups. Publishes a newsletter.

Useful Addresses

Women's Therapy Centre, 6 Manor Gardens, London N7 6LA 01-263 6200 — Runs groups for women. Offers personal counselling and advice.

The Disabled Living Foundation, 380-384 Harrow Road, London W9 2HU 01-289 6111 — Publishes *Disabled Eve: Aids in Menstruation*. Answers individual inquiries on practical solutions to daily living problems caused by disability.

Liberation Network, c/o The Secretary, 68 Aldan House, Duncan Road, London E8 — Information for the disabled woman.

The National Childbirth Trust, 9 Queensborough Terrace, London W2 3TB 01-221 3833 — Provides information on exercises for period problems, relaxation and childbirth.

Action Against Allergy, 43 The Downs, London SW20 8HG 01-947 5082 — Provides information on allergies.

TRANX (National Tranquilliser Advisory Council), 17 Peel Road, Harrow, Middlesex HA3 7QX 01-427 2065 — Offers information and advice regarding problems with tranquillisers and sedatives.

British Migraine Association, 178a High Road, Byfleet, Weybridge, Surrey KT14 7ED 09323 52468 — Provides information about migraine and support for sufferers.

Periods

Endometriosis Society, c/o A. Irving, 65 Holmdene Avenue, Herne Hill, London SE24	Publishes a leaflet on endometriosis and puts sufferers in touch with each other.
Hysterectomy Association, Judy Vaughan, 'Rivendell', Warren Way, Lower Heswall, Wirral L10 9HV 051 342 3167	Counselling for women who have had a hysterectomy. Publishes a leaflet.
Understanding Women, PMT Support Group, Chris Hollick, 6 Hillside Cottages, Leverstock Green, Hemel Hempstead, Herts. 0442 63289	Offers understanding and support to PMT sufferers through personal contact and information.
Katy Gardner, 11 Devonshire Road, Liverpool 8	Answers letters and questions about PMT.
National Association for Premenstrual Syndrome, 23 Upper Park Road, Kingston Upon Thames, Surrey KT2 5LB	National support group for PMT sufferers.
Pre-Menstrual Tension Advisory Service, P.O. Box 268, Hove, East Sussex BN3 1RW 0273 771366	Postal service offering advice on nutritional remedies for premenstrual tension.
Family Planning Information Service, 27-35 Mortimer Street, London W1N 7RJ 01-636 7866	Provides information on family planning and women's health care.